STOP FEELING TIRED!

10 MIND-BODY STEPS TO FIGHT FATIGUE AND FEEL YOUR BEST

GEORGE D. ZGOURIDES, PYS.D.
CHRISTIE S. ZGOURIDES, MA

NEW HARBINGER PUBLICATIONS, INC.

Publisher's Note

Distributed in the U.S.A. by Publishers Group West; in Canada by Raincoast Books; in Great Britain by Hi Marketing, Ltd.; in South Africa by Real Books, Ltd.; in Australia by Boobook; and in New Zealand by Tandem Press.

Copyright © 2003 by George Zgourides and Christie Zgourides
New Harbinger Publications, Inc.
5674 Shattuck Avenue
Oakland, CA 94609

Cover design by Amy Shoup
Cover image by Wilhelm Scholtz/Getty Images
Edited by Carole Honeychurch
Text design by Michele Waters

ISBN 1-57224-313-9 Paperback

New Harbinger Publications' Web site address: www.newharbinger.com

05   04   03

10   9   8   7   6   5   4   3   2   1

First printing

For Galen Mark Eversole, M.D.

CONTENTS

Acknowledgments

Putting a book together requires a great deal of work on the part of many people. We'd especially like to thank Catharine Sutker for her support of this project and Carole Honeychurch for her expert editorial guidance. We'd also like to thank Michele Waters and Amy Shoup for helping to make this book a reality.

INTRODUCTION

Energy is eternal delight.

—William Blake

Let's face it, most Americans today feel worn-out, exhausted, tired, run-down, and used up. We want more energy to enjoy life but can't seem to find an answer to our hectic work schedules, frenzied social demands, constant interruptions, household clutter, and electronic gizmos that don't work when we need them.

Constant fast-paced living, a never-ending push to get ahead, pressing our personal reserves to the limit, and trying to do everything—all of this results in a state of *chronic tiredness*. Millions of us wake up too tired in the morning, load up on coffee and donuts, and drag ourselves from activity to activity throughout the day. If we're lucky, at the end of work we might have just enough strength to grab some fast food on the way home, plop in front of the television, have a couple of drinks, and then toss and turn in bed worrying about everything we didn't get done. Several hours later, it's time to repeat the cycle anew.

No wonder so many Americans are miserable. Tiredness is no fun. It takes the joy out of living. And the reason is obvious. None of us is designed to cope with nonstop fast-paced living. None of us can accomplish absolutely everything we want. When we try, we fall short. As a result of overcommitting and not taking care of ourselves, we end up grumbling about exhaustion, frustration, stress, and health problems, trying to be everything to everyone.

As a therapist, George has found the Eastern view of the phenomenon of everyday tiredness particularly interesting. For example, Oriental medical practitioners refer to a physical, mental, and spiritual state known as *depletion*. We think this is as apt a descriptor as any for lack of pep, and it's one we'll use often in upcoming pages. But suffice it to say for the moment, for us the word "depletion" suggests a *life imbalance characterized by too little energy to live appreciatively and mindfully.*

A Widespread Problem

Without question, many millions of Americans go to their doctor seeking help for persistent feelings of tiredness. These worn-out people know something is wrong but are having trouble identifying exactly what. Understandably, this leads them to seek medical advice. As Ronald L. Hoffman noted in his book, *Tired All the Time: How to Reclaim Your Lost Energy* (1993):

> Americans make a shocking 500 million office visits to doctors every year to complain about generalized fatigue. If the number-one complaint of patients is flu and colds, tiredness is number two. Nearly half of the visitors to my own clinic come because of a mysterious, nonspecific ailment that seems to be ruining their lives: exhaustion. Fatigue has come to be seen as a genuine illness in itself (11).

Yet the answer to their question, "Why am I so tired all the time?" isn't mysterious. According to most Western health experts, tiredness is frequently brought on by factors like stress, excessive weight, unwholesome diet, unrealistic thinking, ineffective coping skills, and too many work and family pressures. Anxiety, depression, a sedentary lifestyle, and an overreliance on medication can also contribute to persistent exhaustion. The bottom line here is: don't feel alone if you're exhausted. Physical-mental exhaustion ranks as one of the most frequent health complaints brought to doctors every year.

Although most of us are run-down from too much stress (which is aggravated by the aforementioned factors, as well as many others), a small percentage of Americans have a diagnosable fatigue disorder, the two most common of which are chronic fatigue syndrome (CFS) and fibromyalgia (described in chapter 1). But even if you don't have a diagnosable, fatigue-related condition, you're tiredness is very real to you. Others, especially the ones making demands on you, may not understand how stressed you are. They could be inclined to take advantage of your good nature, and you suffer.

The personal consequences can be devastating in the long run. For example, too much stress can eventually cause you to experience physical health problems. When stress is the primary culprit, chronic fast-paced activity can lead to any number of disorders, such migraines and stomach hyperacidity. In severe cases, cardiovascular problems can develop.

Even if you're lucky enough to escape medical complications, your stressors and excessive lifestyle still make you unhappy. In fact, you may feel utterly burned out in the worst sense of the term. Does this sound familiar?: you no longer enjoy family relationships and friends; you seclude yourself from coworkers at lunch time; you hate the thought of leaving the house if you don't have to; and you dread one more commitment, even though you're compelled to keep saying yes to those around you—no matter the personal costs. You're miserable, but not quite sure how to free yourself from the merry-go-round of fast living.

Good News for the Weary

Whatever you choose to call it—depletion, tiredness, exhaustion, weariness, fatigue, listlessness, stress, or burnout—a simple, straightforward approach to the imbalances of the American excessive lifestyle is clearly needed. If you're at the point in your own journey that you're reading this book, you've probably already tried various tactics to regain your youthful levels of energy. Vacations haven't worked. Neither have dieting, attending awareness seminars, or complaining. Understandably, you're now ready for a different approach.

We have good news for you. The truth is: *in order to regain lost energy and zest, you must choose to implement those lifestyle changes that'll lead you to simplicity and balance.* And that's why our rallying theme for this book is to *increase your personal energy by reducing stress, improving your lifestyle, and slowing down.*

And why is balance so important? According to Joel Levey and Michele Levey's book, *Living in Balance: A Dynamic Approach for Creating Harmony and Wholeness in a Chaotic World* (1998):

> Though our yearning for balance is a deeply personal quest, it is truly a journey of universal proportions. While at an individual level, we may be feeling overwhelmed with trying to juggle our jobs, family, and PTA, it is helpful to

remember that every thing at every level and dimension of the universe is constantly in search for balance. Indeed, it is the yearning for balance that keeps everything in our universe in motion, while the motion itself provides balance for the dimensions of reality that dwell in stillness (3).

In other words, the search for balance is at the core of our existence. And it has everything to do with your feeling more energetic.

You might also be wondering how finding balance can help you have more energy. As modern-day Americans, we all find ourselves particularly prone to getting out-of-kilter to the point of depleting our overall life-energy reserves (or *Qi*, as the Chinese refer to it). In other words, many of our everyday problems related to tiredness, stress, and general upset are, in reality, the result of being out of balance in other areas of our life. Your goal, at least from our point of view, is to correct your imbalances by attaining and enjoying *just the right amount of energy*—not too little and not too much. In other words, our intent is *not* to teach you how to become even busier than you already are, thus enabling your getting further and further out of balance. Instead, we'll explain how achieving a state of general equilibrium is the most important step in your feeling energized and experiencing life as it's meant to be lived—*intentionally* and *lovingly*. This means choosing as priorities those activities and strategies that contribute to our well being and letting the rest go. Balance also means learning to take time out from our daily busyness for activities that'll invigorate us: eating well, spending time in nature, reading inspirational books, listening to music, reflecting, praying, helping others, and getting lots of sleep, to name just some of the possible steps we might want to try.

Of course, many methods (or steps, as we like to call them), are available to assist you in this process. Borrowing from the best that both Western and Eastern traditions have to offer, we've compiled the most effective and efficient steps to help you develop a more balanced life with the least amount of hassle and disruption to your schedule. Few of us can pack up our bags, hit the road, and move to the proverbial meditative mountain. We can, however, gradually integrate healthful changes into our lives. And as these changes take hold, you'll find you have increased enthusiasm for life, as well as more time to be "in the moment" with yourself and those around you.

What This Book Can Do for You

Given our rather broad professional backgrounds, we have a personal and practical perspective to offer you. We've paid close attention to identifying tried-and-true methods to restore and balance the body's life energy—steps that are approachable but also scientific.

Here we offer you a user-friendly, step-by-step guide for increasing personal energy through physical, mental, and spiritual balance. We build upon integrative medicine concepts that include much self-help information on nutrition, simple living, Oriental medicine, and spirituality as adjuncts to short-term psychological methods for attaining increased energy, health, peace, and overall balance in life.

The chapters of our book build on each other and are organized according to the holistic "biopsychosocial" perspective. That's a fancy way of saying we plan to give biological, psychological, and social recommendations for achieving good physical, mental, and spiritual health. Our goal is to present you with some of the best Eastern and Western programs available for self-enhancement.

We'll give you holistic self-help techniques to increase your quality of life, wellness, happiness, peace, harmony, and quiet—all with aim of your having more pep. We'll also show you how to use the best of Western science and time-proven Eastern energy balancing for renewing your soul, overall health, and life's purpose. Equipped with a combination of mind-body-spirit self-help steps, you'll start on the path to a balanced life in a matter minutes.

Stop Feeling Tired! is divided into three large sections, each of which has engaging chapters focusing on the best, surefire Western, Eastern, and complementary techniques for increasing balance and energy. In part 1, "The Body and Everyday Energy," we'll first define *health psychology* (also known as *mind-body psychology*) and show how it encompasses many helpful views and methods for increasing energy, attaining health, and fostering a loving attitude. We'll look at the biopsychosocial model, which explains psychological and other life phenomena from a holistic point of view. As well, we'll explain some of the main differences between Eastern and Western models of healing, as well as the implications of these differences for self-enhancement and energy restoration. We'll then discuss how such methods as acupressure, acupuncture, herbs, massage, and chiropractic can be useful adjuncts to Western psychological and medical methods. We'll also present information on nutrition, vitamins, herbs, exercise, sleep, and other lifestyle practices.

In part 2, "The Mind and Everyday Energy," we'll recommend psychological self-help techniques that promote energy and balance, with a heavy focus on rational-emotive-behavior therapy (REBT). We'll explain the direct influence that beliefs (thoughts, evaluations, assessments) have on emotions and behaviors as we outline specific, step-by-step REBT procedures for eliminating the kinds of negative self-talk that generates tiredness, burnout, agony, and distress. We'll give practical behavioral advice for improving your overall wellness, including relaxation, visualization, distraction, thought stopping, hypnosis, and biofeedback. We'll also thoroughly explore the role of heightened stress in creating the misery of tiredness and burnout.

Far too often, the spiritual side of life is ignored in favor of drinking alcohol, taking medications, spending more money, accumulating clutter, or socializing. In part 3 of the book, "The Spirit and Everyday Energy," we'll explain how balance isn't easily found without simultaneously working on one's spirituality. We'll have much to say about restoring energy through spiritual balancing, a topic with which you're probably less familiar. We'll also present several methods (for example, prayer, meditation, charitable service) from various spiritual disciplines that are easy to grasp and that provide noticeable, lasting results for yourself and your loved ones.

An Invitation to Change

Our modern, fast-paced world pushes us to our limits. If you're tired of feeling run down and burned out, if you're sick of being in a rut, if you're fed up with stress, we have some great recommendations for you. In *Stop Feeling Tired!*, we give you time-tested, sensible ideas for restoring your energy, vigor, and sense of well being naturally.

Imagine, perhaps for the first time in years, waking up eager to face the new day with all its challenges. Imagine feeling wide awake all afternoon without needing to take a nap or guzzle an extra cup of coffee. Imagine coming home from work, enjoying a wholesome dinner, having fun with your children and pets, and getting a restful night's sleep.

All of this and more is possible when you decide to accept our invitation to approach life in a new way. But please don't forget: *change requires effort*. Nothing worthwhile in life is easy or fast. Making the kinds of life-altering changes needed to reclaim lost passion is tough. There are no magic pills or wands that'll solve your problems. We all know this from personal experience.

Nor can anyone else make needed changes for you. It's totally up to you. *You* have to decide to make the necessary changes. *You* have to decide when enough is enough. *You* have to say no to excesses of modern living. Put simply, *you have to decide to take responsibility for transforming your own life*. No one else is going to help you find inner happiness. The ball is in your court!

Whether you're overcommitted, overrun, overworked, or all of the above, *Stop Feeling Tired!* can be a wonderful first step to changing your life from a daily struggle with tiredness to a daily adventure with energy, love, and wellness.

FEATURE: SELF-HELP ENERGY?

We're often asked why we so strongly support self-help materials. The answer is quite simple: we believe everyone should have access to information that can help bring about positive changes. A book like this one, which is much less expensive than personal-growth counseling or a weekend retreat, is easily available. It's an excellent first step for self-enhancement. And that's why we've written *Stop Feeling Tired!* We want you to have the necessary tools for helping yourself feel better through finding balance in your life. Remember, there's little in life that's as empowering as your being able to take charge and work to resolve your own problems.

We think of self-help as a form of deliberate self-coping. In other words, each time you make plans, imagine a better way, weigh alternatives, or solve problems, you're engaging in self-helping behavior. And we believe you can learn to handle your own distressing situations with a conscious decision to improve yourself. You can learn to alter your own feelings, thoughts, and actions. You can learn to identify your own personal flaws and decide to become the master of your circumstances.

This isn't to say you must always go it alone. Whenever feasible, you should seek support from those around you. And there might be times when it's good to seek professional assistance; there's no shame in asking for help. But much of the time you can help yourself without the cost and expense of seeing a psychologist or counselor. Self-help, then, becomes self-improvement, self-responsibility, and self-reliance.

If the idea of helping yourself overcome your tiredness sounds impractical, know you're not the only one who thinks this way. After all, today's society encourages us to seek to be changed by others rather seeking to change ourselves. That's why we end up feeling bullied by others, situations, or whatever. And then we feel incapable of developing our coping skills or solving our problems.

But this need not be so. A peaceful and energized life, while requiring plenty of motivation and hard work on your part, is certainly within your grasp. You can do it! You need only choose to reflect on your life in a fresh way.

PART 1

THE BODY AND EVERYDAY ENERGY

CHAPTER 1

ENERGIZE YOURSELF WITH HEALTH PSYCHOLOGY

We are used to the actions of human beings, not to their stillness.

—V. S. Pritchett

Do any of these remarks sound familiar?

"I'm so tired I can't see straight."

"I go and go and go all day, and most nights I've got just enough energy to fall asleep in front of the TV."

"If one more thing breaks down around our house, I think I'll scream!"

"I'm really tired of trying to be the ultimate soccer mom."

"I work so many long hours during the week that I'm practically worthless by Saturday."

"The thought of taking on one more task makes me sick!"

If you ever have thoughts like these, we'd like to welcome you to the club! Just like us, you and millions of other Americans know what it means to be chronically tired. In fact, excessive tiredness is one of the most frequent health complaints in the United States today.

If you're wondering why everyone around you seems fed up, run down, and exhausted, the answer isn't all that mysterious. *Americans are overworked, overcommitted, overspent, and overweight.* These four "Big O's" might sound obvious, but we all know deep-down that they're true.

A Definition

And what exactly is chronic tiredness or fatigue? We especially like the way Charles Kuntzleman defined it in *Maximizing Your Energy and Personal Productivity* (1992):

> Chronic fatigue, simply stated, is a pervasive feeling of a total shortage of energy. If you're able to function at all, it is only due to an immense effort of the will. You feel as though the force of gravity has doubled when it comes to getting out of bed in the morning. Relationships seem to require more effort than they're worth. Your job is like a dead weight. You wonder why you've stayed with it so long. Your very shoes seem to have rubber cement gumming up their soles, holding you back. A tremendous amount of willpower must be mustered to do anything out of a daily routine of things. And even the daily routine can get to be too much. How many times have you thought, "I'm too tired to get off the couch and crawl into bed"? That's chronic fatigue.
>
> People who suffer this type of chronic fatigue are from all socioeconomic classes. They include corporate ladder climbers, decision makers, custodians, teachers, ministers, housewives, truck drivers, doctors, students, and so forth. They find themselves physically and emotionally bankrupt. Their brains seem to have wilted and all body functions have gone limp with it (12).

And on the topic of why we're all so frustrated and burned out, consider these words from Richard Carlson's book, *Don't Sweat the Small Stuff ... and It's All Small Stuff* (1997):

We lose sight of the bigger picture, focus on the negative, and annoy other people who might otherwise help us. In short, we live our lives as if they were one great big emergency! We often rush around looking busy, trying to solve problems, but in reality, we are often compounding them. Because everything seems like such a big deal, we end up spending our lives dealing with one drama after another (1).

These descriptions of American's hyperactivity and chronic fatigue nail our point on the head! *Too much activity means too little energy.* So, for us, the type of tiredness we're describing in this book is the everyday sort that results from staying too busy, not taking care of ourselves, and not properly handling our stress.

Everyday tiredness is a lack of personal energy that results when life gets out-of-balance. Each day becomes nothing more than a wearisome attempt to make it through yet another battle. If it isn't family or school, it's work, kids, neighbors, errands, or something else. People pull at us from every direction. We try to say no, but they pester us until we relent. In the end, we feel this inner need to push ourselves harder and harder, while at the same time society also pressures us to go faster and faster. Let's face it, this sort of I-give-and-you-take relationship is very unhealthy.

Bigger, Faster, Better, Newer

We've noticed two disturbing trends in recent decades: 1. increasing societal expectations that we do everything instantly and perfectly, and 2. cultural pressure that we keep up with the latest of everything. "More, more, and still more" has become the modern American theme.

The demands of modern life place great strain on us all, which means most of us have a daily battle of one sort or another to wage. We spend countless hours at jobs requiring perfect reports that are "due yesterday." And our work has become even more demanding as corporate employers combine jobs at the bottom to save money.

We get especially annoyed over everyday hassles when nothing is accomplished. For example, your credit-card payment gets lost in the mail, so you get socked with a twenty-nine-dollar late charge. Then you try to get through to a customer "no-service" representative (as consumer advocate Clark Howard calls these people) to complain, only to become hopelessly lost in a telephone menu that won't let you talk to a human being. Then your office fax breaks down when you absolutely need it to work. So, you call a repair person, who charges you top dollar for a service call but can't get the machine fixed. At the end of your day, you still have a late charge on your credit-card statement, and your fax is still broken.

A continuous bombardment of advertisements—radio, television, billboards, e-mail spam—convince us to compete for the good life (whatever that's supposed to be). Then we're caught in the cycle of buying the latest slick SUV, DVD player, PDA, or computer every time the old one goes "obsolete." After all, we *must* keep up with all the newest technology, right?

Even our children succumb. They, too, want the latest video games and computer toys. They also expect to be on the go, busy, and entertained constantly. One or two extracurricular activities aren't enough; parents are required to be "hyper-parents" and drive their kids all over town most every afternoon. These same parents feel guilty if they don't provide their children with every opportunity (and more) that's available out there. What ever happened to children reading or playing outside with their neighborhood friends?

Then there are the telemarketers who continually interrupt us at mealtime. "Buy our product." "Take advantage of our great offer . . . available only today." "Open a credit-card account with us." Pressure, pressure, and more pressure. It can be maddening!

We can't even sit at home and quietly watch television. Broadcast commercials keep getting louder and bolder, not to mention that we have to decide which of 160 cable channels and hundreds of programs to watch. *There are so many choices today that it's becoming increasingly difficult for Americans to stay calm, focused, and balanced.*

The Whys and Wherefores

We could blame today's situation on money. After all, capitalism encourages the four "Big O's": *overworking, overcommitting, overspending,* and *overeating.* But the problem goes far beyond money and external pressure. At the heart of the Big O's is internal pressure—our unrealistic need to look busy, feel accepted by those around us, and satisfy our own needs, regardless of what our actions do to our bodies or the environment. That's right, a lot of us connect our self-acceptance and self-esteem to our accomplishments and attainments, including how others see us and how much stuff we can own. As a good friend of ours described:

> For many years I simultaneously taught college full-time as an art instructor and served as a minister at my church. To make ends meet, I've also held different part-time jobs, including

writing ad copy for our local paper. This is in addition to being married, raising two kids, and keeping two dogs. I didn't seem to have trouble juggling everything when I was younger, but now that I'm over forty I'm just not as motivated. Either the demands have increased, or I'm more exhausted. Or, maybe it's both. Either way, I feel burned out. I don't seem to want to do much of anything now unless I absolutely have to. But, the funny thing is, when my schedule lightens up, I end up getting myself into more projects. It's sort of like, I'm a hard-working, good person if I'm busy, but I'm a lazy, bad person if I'm not. That's why I can't let myself have any free time. It's taken me some time and lots of thinking to come to the conclusion that I'm my own worst enemy.

If this rings true for you, you're one of many millions of Americans who dislike the hectic life of the twenty-first century but keep taking on more and more responsibilities. That's right. If you're tired all the time, you're probably causing most of your own problems, even if you don't realize it.

We're here to remind you that you can regain normal energy and move on with enjoying your life. *Enough really can be enough!* You really can let go of all those "hyper's" in your life!

It's up to you to make the changes, though. The first step is understanding what the basic problem is.

Stress and Imbalance

Chronic tiredness doesn't just appear out of nowhere; it's the end result of a series of events in your life. In a nutshell, all of your life pressures, demands, and poor habits add up to a nasty negative: *too much stress*, both mentally and physically. This stress leads to an energy imbalance, which, in turn, leads to chronic tiredness. It's that straightforward.

Of course, we all have different internal and external pressures in life, so the causes of our individual stress will be different, too. But the result is usually the same if you haven't learned to effectively handle your stress: persistent tiredness that won't let up.

We've made of point of emphasizing just how powerful stress can be in making you feel tired all the time. Why? Some estimates are that as many as 75 percent of all visits to physicians are for stress-related problems. This alarming statistic alone should indicate the need for health psychologists to continue studying the role of stress in diverse physical conditions, including migraines, hypertension, immune disorders like AIDS, and even cancer. Information gleaned from this type of research should prove useful in figuring out which mind-body approaches are the best antidotes to stress.

As we mentioned in the introduction to *Stop Feeling Tired!*, stress has a unique role in creating tiredness. This makes sense, because stress alters general perceptions and interpretations of your life. When under stress, you probably react more ineffectively to life's hassles. This inefficiency then brings about imbalance, which then drains away your energy. The stress causes imbalance, which causes less energy, which causes more stress. And so the cycle goes.

This means the answer is to eliminate stress, right? Not exactly. Stress is unavoidable; if you have no stress at all, you're not alive. Technically, it's not the amount or type of stress that makes the difference; it's how you handle whatever stress you have. This is why we can safely argue that *ineffective coping* is at the heart of what causes excessive stress for most of us.

In our opinion (and we'll have more to say about this in later chapters), stress, imbalance, and everyday tiredness usually come from and are worsened by a person's *irrational thoughts* and *unhealthy behaviors*. (Our use of the word "irrational" should be taken to mean "unrealistic." We don't mean it as an insult or put down!) Put another way, although numerous causes like stress and pent-up emotions play leading roles in creating the energy imbalances that trigger chronic tiredness, *everyday tiredness mostly has to do with the way you think about and approach your life and health*. The good news, of course, is that you can do something about your chronic tiredness because *you can change your thinking and behavior*.

We'll have lots to say about stress, its causes, and its remedies throughout this book. But we'd like to take a few moments here to explain the role that energy imbalance plays in chronic tiredness.

Yin and Yang

In ancient times, Chinese physicians were also philosophers firmly grounded in the Taoist tradition. The Tao emphasizes a special harmony in the nature of all things, including the human body.

From the perspective of Traditional Chinese Medicine (TCM), your physical, mental, and spiritual health is intimately related to the ability of your body's life energy, or *Qi* (pronounced "chee"), to flow freely. More accurately, *Qi* is thought to be living energy that flows through your body along pathways called *meridians*. Too little *Qi* available for use in the body results in a state of being known as *depletion*, which Westerners might describe with such words as "used up," "burned out," or "run down."

Qi is also said to manifest itself in the body (as well as the rest of creation) as two opposing yet complementary qualities: *Yin* and *Yang*. *Yin* and *Yang* represent such aspects as cold (*Yin*) and hot (*Yang*), wet (*Yin*) and dry (*Yang*), night (*Yin*) and day (*Yang*), as well as many other opposing but complementary conditions.

The harmony of health especially depends on the balance of *Yin* and *Yang*. Because humans are in dynamic balance with other aspects of nature, we constantly respond to external and internal influences in an attempt to maintain balance. When we don't adapt, we go out of balance and develop sickness. The purpose of a TCM diagnosis is to identify this imbalance.

When *Yin* and *Yang* are harmoniously balanced and *Qi* flows smoothly, health and energy are at their fullest potential. This means to protect your *Qi* and restore your lost energy, you have to find balance in your life. In TCM, the primary goal is to prevent imbalance and its consequences—disease, misery, fatigue, and so forth. In other words, ailments of most every type are the consequences of the imbalance of *Qi*. Treatments like acupuncture, massage, diet, herbal remedies, exercise, controlled breathing, lifestyle changes, mindfulness, and meditation are prescribed to restore lost balance and assist you in achieving a healthy, balanced life.

Of course, it's impossible to give an adequate review of thousands of years of Oriental philosophy and medicine in these few pages. Hopefully, the concepts mentioned here will give you at least a couple of new insights into your life, and inspire you to read more about TCM.

The Mind-Body Connection

It's easier to relax while on a beach in the Caribbean than in the midst of work and family hassles. Who can possibly be their best, for example, when they're overworked, loaded up on caffeine and sugar, or depressed? We all know that the daily stresses of life—whatever the source—drain our physical energy to the point that even a simple nuisance, like a broken traffic light, can be enough to send us over the edge. You don't have to be a detective to see how the human mind and body are connected in some marvelous ways.

From a Western perspective, tiredness is fundamentally a "mind-body" problem. In other words, most clinicians in this country see everyday tiredness as including both physical and mental components, meaning it generally isn't a purely medical problem. (There are exceptions: some serious medical disorders like diabetes have exhaustion as a primary symptom.) Sometimes your tiredness is more mental than physical, and sometimes more physical than mental. But there is always a connection between the two, even though the mental part (for example, your decisions about your lifestyle) probably plays a larger role in your experience of everyday tiredness.

Sadly, there are many social stigmas associated with anything "mental." And not surprisingly, those of you who experience everyday tiredness, as a group, probably don't welcome the idea of a psychological label. You may see any hint that you could suffer from stress or make poor lifestyle decisions as insulting. In fact, it may be easier for you to have an official medical diagnosis, which implies your tiredness is somehow more "real" or "legitimate" than not. For you, having a psychological issue could seem akin to having a personal weakness or moral defect. While utterly untrue, our culture fosters this type of nonsense. If you're moral and strong, you're supposed to be able to solve your own problems. These kinds of irrational notions can become the source of your "blind spot"—denial of the role that psychological factors play in your difficulties, which also means denial of your potential role in your own recovery. Please remember that you're not lazy, immoral, or weak in any way because stress has gotten the best of you.

What is Health Psychology?

Questions concerning the relation between the body and mind are nothing new and are not of sole interest to modern Americans. The issue has piqued the curiosity of philosophers and scientists for millennia.

Consider philosophy and psychology (which prior to 1879 were generally considered to be one and the same). Great thinkers from these disciplines have historically described *mind-body dualism*, which implies that the mind and body are distinct forms of unrelated matter. For this reason, a "dualist" might disapprove of any assumption that equates the human mind with the physical mechanism of the brain.

More recent views on this topic are based, at least in part, on the writings of seventeenth-century French mathematician and philosopher Rene Descartes. With his famous phrase, *"Cogito, ergo sum"* (Latin, meaning "I think, therefore I am"), Descartes described the mind as an immaterial substance that engages in the activities of thinking, reasoning, and imagining. He also described the mind as being completely separate from the rest of the body. Among the problems with dualism as a concept is its inability to define precisely what a mental substance, or "essence," actually is. Many such criticisms have led modern theorists to abandon dualism for scientific approaches to the mind-body connection.

Today's scientists have become increasingly fascinated with the idea that our thoughts, emotions, behaviors, and health are all interdependent. Their interest has led to a new branch of psychology known as *health psychology* (also known as *mind-body psychology, behavioral medicine,* or *psychosomatic medicine*), as well as a new branch of medicine known as *psychoneuroimmunology*. Of these two broad categories, health psychology is the more inclusive in its study of mind-body-spirit events, while psychoneuroimmunology is more specific in its study of the links between emotions and the immune system.

An important goal of health psychologists is to understand the role that mental factors play in overall health. Mind-body psychologists typically study why people become sick, how their behavior influences their health, and how they keep free of illness. Health psychologists are especially interested in how stress affects the brain and other body structures, and vice versa. They are also interested in various mind-body problems in which physical symptoms appear almost exclusively in response to psychological factors. (This is in contrast to the physical conditions and diseases that are that are *worsened* by psychological factors, but not *caused* by them.)

Health psychologists study many other health-related topics, such as the promotion of fitness, instruction in stress management, and the enhancement of health-care policies and services, to name just a couple of topics.

And the Significance?

The interdependence of the mind and body is central to the premise of this book: that your feelings of physical tiredness are related to your mental and spiritual approach to life. Of course, the mind-body connection extends far beyond ordinary tiredness. It's evident in everything we do, from enjoying music, to sending an e-mail, to mastering an academic subject in school. In fact, it's difficult *not* to find these links in our lives. However, the same mind-body interactions that bring us joy in life also pose special problems, as is the case with persistently tired people.

The answer to chronic tiredness, then, is clear. You need to intervene at the levels of mind, body, and spirit. Specifically, simplifying your life and changing your thinking will reduce your stress, which will reduce your *Qi* imbalance, which will reduce your chronic tiredness.

In short, most health psychologists would agree that *virtually all mind-body problems—whether they're more physical or more mental—respond to self-help strategies that simplify life, reduce stress, and alter ineffective thinking patterns.*

This emphasis on interrelations among your thoughts, emotions, and behaviors means *you can choose to make a difference in your recovery from chronic tiredness.* It means that by changing the way you look at your world, you can influence the course of your life. We'll speak more to this process of reframing your perceptions and attitudes—a process termed *cognitive restructuring*—in chapter 5.

Harmony and Balance

We've already noted several topics that health psychologists emphasize: promoting health, identifying mental factors in disease, improving health care, and so on. Another popular trend in health psychology is to teach effective personal attitudes and behaviors that contribute to positive physical and mental health. Not surprisingly, this approach is perfectly applicable to cases of everyday tiredness.

Four broad areas for helping you restore balance and alleviate chronic tiredness are exercise, nutrition, attitude, and spirituality. These and numerous other balance-related topics will be discussed in greater detail in upcoming chapters.

Exercise

Most Americans today are aware of the many advantages of aerobic exercise for good health. Walking, running, jogging, swimming, cycling, dancing, and cross-country skiing increase oxygen consumption, particularly when sustained for a minimum of fifteen to thirty minutes three or more times per week. The net result is conditioning of both respiratory and coronary systems that leads to such health benefits as weight control, cardiovascular fitness, and regulation of cholesterol and glucose levels. Health psychology research further indicates that exercise decreases stress and restores personal energy.

Even though the vast majority of people know the advantages of aerobic exercise, only about half who start an exercise program continue past six months. Accordingly, health psychologists strive to improve people's compliance with their exercise programs. Why? Research studies suggest that having definable goals (for example, losing fifteen pounds of fat) and a positive attitude improves the chances that you'll stick to an exercise schedule long-term.

We explain how exercise can give you balanced energy in more detail in the next chapter.

Nutrition

The adage "You are what you eat" rings truer than most of us care to admit. Our overall diet strongly affects our physical and mental health. This is one reason why health psychologists look for ways to assist persons in strengthening their health through sound nutrition. Little doubt remains that certain food items bring about and aggravate certain conditions. As one example, excessive intake of salt is often related to hypertension, and foods high in fat are often related to high cholesterol.

Simple carbohydrates—like those found in sweets—are quickly digested and provide you with an energy rush. Unfortunately, they also lack the essential nutrients needed for long-term energy and frequently cause a crash that makes you crave more sweets. The result? Overconsumption of sweets high in calories, which can lead to tiredness. Too much sugar in your diet can also cause health problems like obesity, diabetes, dental cavities, and anxiety disorders. Simple carbohydrates may be useful for immediate energy (for example, during times of exertion), but they shouldn't be a cornerstone of your diet. If you find yourself consuming a great deal of sugar (as well as caffeine or alcohol) throughout the day just to keep yourself moving, you need to make some changes if you want to feel energetic. Think about eating lots of complex carbohydrates like those found in whole-grain bread and pasta. These are slowly digested and produce sustained levels of energy. Complex carbohydrates should make up the largest percentage of calories that you eat each day.

The amino acid L-Carnitine and such vitamins as pantothenic acid (B5) increase energy production in your body. And several herbs like ginseng and ginko are thought to do the same. Keep in mind that opinions with respect to vitamins and herbs vary considerably across disciplines and even clinicians, so you'll have to be the judge of what works best for you. We'll have much more to say about nutrition in chapter 3.

Attitude

Crucial to our entire program for *Stop Feeling Tired!* is eliminating your cognitive distortions, or the irrational thoughts that keep you from enjoying a more zestful and loving life. Cognitive psychology, which we explain in detail in chapter 5, teaches you how ineffective thinking patterns cause most of your problems. The idea is for you to learn to challenge your distorted views of life that are prompting you into ill-chosen actions. For example, if you incorrectly think you need to say yes to everyone else's requests even when you're already over-committed, attitudinal reframing can help you say no by teaching you to dispute your irrational assumptions of having to please others. Cognitive therapy gives you some very powerful tools for stopping stress and getting your hectic life back in balance.

Spirituality

Ask most anyone who is religious, and they'll tell you that good health is absolutely related to spirituality and its fruits, which include peace, love, self-acceptance, faith, hope, responsibility, joy, openness, empathy, charity, and service to others. We'll have more to say about the role of spirituality in overcoming everyday tiredness in chapters 9 and 10. But suffice it to say for the moment, it's helpful to know that many people are victorious over exhaustion as they begin to work on their spiritual awareness and growth.

A Word of Caution

This book is primarily for people with everyday tiredness from too much stress, bad lifestyle choices, failure to say no, and so on. However, there are cases when fatigue and exhaustion are actual physical disorders. While the suggestions we offer in this book certainly won't hurt you if you have a medical diagnosis for your tiredness, you must be under the care of a licensed health-care professional and have him or her give you the go ahead to follow our suggestions. Medical conditions don't usually respond well to self-help treatments unless these are used as adjuncts to regular medical care. And tiredness can be a symptom of many medical problems, some of them quite serious (for example, thyroid problems, diabetes, cardiovascular disease, multiple sclerosis, sleep disorders, depression). This means you must have yourself checked out by a physician or nurse to determine if your tiredness is medical, lifestyle-related, or something else. We can't remind you enough that *self-diagnosis is a recipe for disaster.*

Of course, when you're battling exhaustion, you probably feel like you've got a serious disease, even if you don't. And you'd probably take some comfort in thinking you've got an official, diagnosable condition rather than an ineffective coping style. Why do we find it easier to accept a medical disease over a psychological issue? People like nice, neat labels. Unfortunately, life usually isn't so straightforward. We live in a medicalized society that wants to label all bothersome emotional problems as bona fide diseases. Doing this seems to lessen people's guilt or shame over having psychological issues, as well as eliminate the pressure they might feel to resolve their own problems.

Let's face it, if it's "diagnosable," then it's somehow more legitimate. And the implication is there must be a quick-fix answer available somewhere, if only the right specialist, medicine, or technique can be found.

In Conclusion

Health psychology is a scientific discipline devoted to exploring how closely interrelated the human mind and body are. Hopefully, we've made the case in this chapter that a good deal of everyday tiredness comes from your being out of balance in response to the daily stresses of life.

Everyday tiredness exists at the level of the mind-body interface and is a true reflection of how the mind and body can work together for both good and bad. From both Eastern and Western perspectives, chronic tiredness is traceable to an out-of-balance lifestyle, which is linked to stress, unhealthy eating habits, a sedentary lifestyle, negative attitude, and lack of interest in spiritual matters. But whatever its cause, feeling burned out is tough! That's why we've written this book—to provide you with an integrative, step-by-step plan for balancing your personal energy for better physical, mental, and spiritual health.

Our good news, of course, is that you can do something about your life being out-of-balance. And in choosing to do so, you'll reap the rewards of renewed health, vigor, and everyday energy.

FEATURE:
TWO EXHAUSTING CONDITIONS

While there are a variety of medical conditions that include tiredness as a symptom, two of the most common in which tiredness is the central feature are *fibromyalgia syndrome* (FMS) and *chronic fatigue syndrome* (CFS). Both have received increased attention from the medical community in recent years, although many clinicians continue to question the validity of FMS and CFS as medical diagnoses. Our purpose isn't to make a case one way or the other for either of these syndromes; rather, we present some basic information for your personal use.

Fibromyalgia Syndrome

FMS is a musculoskeletal pain and fatigue disorder characterized by chronic exhaustion, body aches, painful "trigger points" (small painful areas), depression, irritable bowel, headaches, and sleep disturbances—symptoms that occur to such a degree that patients become disabled. Acknowledged as a legitimate diagnosis by the National Institute of Health (NIH), FMS afflicts an estimated five million of all Americans, the common onset of symptoms occurring between the ages of thirty-five and sixty years-old (Fransen and Russell 1996). FMS was previously termed *fibrositis*, which implied the presence of an inflammation in the muscles.

Researchers don't agree on what causes FMS, although many believe sufferers are genetically predisposed. They also think excess stress, infection, or other events can trigger the disease. Other researchers argue that malfunctions within the central nervous system (for example, abnormal levels of neurotransmitters and/or hormones) cause FMS. Changes in weather, cold or drafty environments, hormonal fluctuations (premenstrual and menopausal states), stress, depression, anxiety, and overexertion can all contribute to symptom flare-ups.

Whatever its cause, FMS is frequently dismissed as "psychosomatic" or misdiagnosed as the flu, arthritis, or other inflammatory disease. Sometimes, doctors incorrectly use FMS as a kind of "wastebasket" diagnosis when they can't figure out what's wrong with a patient. Treatments are traditionally geared toward reducing pain and improving the quality of sleep.

Chronic Fatigue Syndrome

CFS is a complicated and incapacitating chronic disorder that affects the brain and numerous body systems. Symptoms often include debilitating fatigue, lack of stamina, poor short-term memory, and difficulty concentrating. CFS also occurs with flu-like symptoms, including profound pain in the muscles and joints, sore throat, tender lymph nodes, headaches, and poor sleep. As many as 800,000 Americans suffer from CFS (Jason et al. 1999).

For many years, clinicians thought CFS resulted from the Epstein-Barr Virus (EBV), which is the virus that causes mononucleosis. But scientific research has not borne this theory out. Instead, the possible causes of CFS appear to be many. According to the Centers for Disease Control (CDC 2002) Web site, some of the more researched possibilities include viral infection, traumatic conditions, toxins, and stress.

Although its actual causes remain unknown, CFS requires regular medical visits. Treatments might include medications, vitamin supplements, herbs, exercises, and counseling.

CHAPTER 2

CONSIDERING THE WHOLE PICTURE: HOLISM AND YOU

Slow and steady wins the race.

—Aesop

Our discussion so far of balance, energy, and the mind-body connection is, in essence, a discussion of *holism*, which is a way of looking at the world from many different perspectives. More and more, health psychologists are acknowledging the fact that life must be considered from more than one point of view. Let's face it, life is quite complicated, so to reduce life events to a single explanation is just too simplistic (or reductionistic). Any perspective that combines body, mind, and spirit is a holistic perspective. Those behaviors that build upon a holistic perspective to help you find balance in life are known collectively as *holistic lifestyle practices*—the approach we prefer to take for restored pep and gusto.

Your starting point for a more holistic lifestyle is awareness that attitudes and behaviors greatly affect your health, either positively or negatively, depending on your choices. If you want to find harmony and peace while reducing the stresses that zap your energy, you need to have a strong commitment to doing what's in the best interest of your physical, mental, and spiritual health.

Let's consider an example of applying our holistic model to everyday tiredness. Some people find it difficult or impossible to be assertive around other people. And in taking on every demand that comes their way, these folks quickly become burned out as a result of not setting clear limits or boundaries. This lack of assertion can be the result of any of a number of causes, but most often comes from *injunctions*, or early childhood messages, revolving around the need for others' approval. You may have been given the message that you should be "seen and not heard," and that it's wrong to inconvenience others by expressing your needs. Many of us receive irrational or conflicting messages about assertiveness from our family, teachers, friends, pastors, and the media. Knowing which system gave what message can be both enlightening and helpful for challenging these messages.

Moreover, for those of us raised in a religious environment, the teachings, morals, and values set forth by organized religion can also play a powerful role, be it healthy or harmful. For example, some religious groups teach that it's necessary to do more and more to either obtain God's favor, or to prove you still have God's favor. Unfortunately, both of these approaches to spirituality ignore the role that God's freely given grace plays in our lives.

As a real-life example of our holistic model (with applicable perspectives appearing in parentheses), Bill thinks of himself as an overly nice guy who was raised to believe that if you're good you must always help others and "go the extra mile" (mental). As Bill obsesses over needing to be a good Christian, he refuses to turn anyone down, no matter how absurd their request for help is (mental). Bill spends so many hours volunteering at his church and putting in "freebie" hours on the job that he becomes distracted from fully immersing himself in his family life (social). In time, his nervous system becomes so aroused that relaxing and even sleeping become difficult, which causes his stress levels to continue to rise (physical). Bill becomes more and more exhausted, and when he can't concentrate on his job or anything else, he tries harder and harder to compensate by consuming inordinate amounts of sugar and caffeine (physical). Meanwhile, he worries more and more about not measuring up (mental), so he volunteers even more and begins demanding that his family attend church several times a week. This pressure inadvertently creates a hostile home environment that further contributes to Bill's troubles (social). This cycle continues to the point that Bill becomes so exhausted that his health begins to deteriorate (physical).

Get the idea? Bill doesn't present a simple cause-and-effect predicament. He has multiple issues—mental, physical, and social—all of which interact to create a tough challenge. Considering the entire picture of Bill's predicament, a counselor might choose to help Bill by first treating his most noticeable issues—in this case, his distorted thinking about feeling adequate—followed by treating the rest of his problems.

One final consideration related to everyday tiredness involves benefits that become attached to the exhausted role within a family or other social system. In other words, tiredness can occasionally function as a coping mechanism that relieves sufferers of some responsibility (for example, "I'm exhausted, so I can't fix the fence this afternoon.") The "out," or relief of responsibility this provides, is called a secondary gain. *Secondary gain* refers to the benefit you get by reacting in ways that sustain your problems, usually by reinforcing them; basically, you receive some indirect reward from staying tired. Examples include attention from family members, financial incentives, and avoidance of undesirable situations. This is in contrast to *primary gain*, in which your problems directly satisfy some psychological need or conflict. Here your tiredness serves an important psychological purpose and resolves a conflict that you might not otherwise be able to handle. Both secondary and primary gains can be present in cases of chronic fatigue.

If you suffer from everyday tiredness, you'd best not ignore the role that secondary gain may play in your continuing to be overly run down.

Holistic Practices

In this section, we examine important holistic lifestyle practices that'll help rebalance your life for more energy and a renewed sense of vitality.

Enjoying Fresh Air and Nature

In our daily routines, most of us go from house to car to work, barely stepping outside. Some of us may go from house to garage to parking garage to work without ever looking up to see the sky. Perhaps it only gets our attention when it rains on us—or, in dry years, when it fails to do so. The only thought we may give the outdoors is how it'll affect our plans—that is, will it rain on the kids' soccer game today?

Most Americans live either in urban or suburban areas: city apartments with no yard or maybe only a four-by-six-foot "balcony" or "patio," a token nod to the need for fresh air and sunshine. Often suburban homes sit on small lots with postage-stamp-sized yards. Indeed, in some neighborhoods homes are now being built so closely together, one of our friends jokes that contractors could save money by putting in a single gutter between two houses and letting both roofs drain into it. While we commend building practices that reduce urban and suburban sprawl, we must also take into account how this affects us as the folks who live there, and find ways to bring our lives back into balance.

From the beginning of modern humanity (thousands of years ago) until the Industrial Revolution (barely two hundred years ago), human beings lived in close proximity to and at the mercy of nature. In those thousands of years of human development and experience, humans developed a mind-body-spirit need for nature.

As we've advanced from an agrarian to an industrial to service/office society, we've moved ever farther from our natural environment. And, in so doing, we lose focus on who we are and where we are in relation to the rest of the world. The pace and focus of our lives makes our vision ever more egocentric and detached from the natural environment. The ultimate consequence is separation from ourselves.

It's also interesting that as our culture moves farther and farther from nature, as we spend more hours on the Internet or watching TV instead of involved in backyard or other outdoor activities, the food we eat becomes equally unnatural. As we distance ourselves from where the food is grown or raised, as we've increasingly eaten manufactured and prepared foods, we've begun to forget what much of our food used to taste like. Chicken is a prime example of what we mean.

Growing up in rural Oregon, Christie had the benefit of eating farm-fresh vegetables, eggs, and chickens. She knows what a farm-raised chicken tastes like, and it bears little resemblance to the steroid, corn-fed, monster-sized chicken breasts that now populate the modern grocery shelf. If more people knew what a real chicken tastes like, they'd be less inclined to say that exotic food "tastes like chicken." And this isn't just Christie's experience. We once had a student from Japan who complained one day that American chicken had "no taste." The other students dismissed his comment with the observation that chicken just doesn't have much taste. The Japanese student protested that Japanese chickens do and revealed in the course of the conversation that his grandmother raised the chickens they ate. We informed him that the difference wasn't American versus Japanese chickens, but farm-fresh, natural versus commercially raised chickens.

In our modern urban and suburban worlds, we're so far removed from the natural world that most of us don't even know what it tastes, smells, or looks like anymore. In our ever-more artificial environments, our loss of connection to the natural world is killing us, stressful artificial moment by stressful artificial moment. You might consider if the food we eat were closer to old-fashioned farm fresh, how much easier it might be to eat healthy foods and avoid the junk.

When average Americans do attempt to "get back to nature," they often do so with the convenience of the American living room: a camper with refrigerator, TV reception, and a queen-sized bed. While RVs may be a great way to see the world in retirement, they're not usually the best way to encounter the natural world. We can't escape our artificiality if we take it with us.

Are we suggesting a seven-day backpack trip in the wilderness? No, even though that might not hurt. The goal here is to raise awareness about how far removed we are from our natural world and the consequences of that distance. Taking time to become more aware of and connected to our natural world is but one part (a vital part) of rebalancing our total lives and taking one more crucial step in claiming the energy that's ours.

Activity and Exercise

Regular physical activity is important for good health in people of all ages. In fact, since the publication of the U.S. Department of Health and Human Services' *Healthy People 2000: National Health Promotion and Disease Prevention* (1992), a recognized goal in this country has been to increase participation in physical activity for all persons. Specifically, experts recommend that adults exercise (or engage in other rigorous physical activity) for a minimum of thirty minutes daily or as often as possible for cardiovascular benefits (Troiano, Macera, and Ballard-Barbash 2001). To reduce the risk of certain cancers, the American Cancer Society has published guidelines that require even more exercise. According to the April 2002 issue of *CA: A Cancer Journal for Clinicians*:

> Current evidence suggests that there is substantial risk reduction for colon cancer from simply not being sedentary. And by participating in moderate-to-vigorous physical activity at least 45 minutes on five or more days of the week, individuals may achieve optimal activity levels needed to reduce the risk of developing both breast and colon cancers,

as well as several other types of cancer, including kidney, endometrial, and esophageal cancer (Byers et al. 2002, 99).

Understandably, many physicians and researchers are concerned that these goals are not being reached by most Americans, but especially older Americans (National Institute on Aging 2002).

We all know that increasing levels of physical activity increases aerobic capacity, reduces obesity, and increases self-esteem—all of which can even help reduce your chances of dying early. We know we need to exercise, yet most of us don't. Or, we do for a while, then we slip back into old, idle habits. Most Americans have purchased some kind of exercise or fitness equipment, always with the best of intentions, only to have it end up in the garage or storage closet. On a sunny afternoon walk through our neighborhood, we can't help but notice the open garage doors revealing neatly folded treadmills, weight-lifting contraptions, stair steppers, and a vast array of other equipment—all quiet testimonials to the good intentions and failed actions of their owners. Most fitness equipment is advertised as folding neatly for storage, a feature probably used more than whatever the original purpose of the equipment might have been.

Then there are the untold stacks of aerobic, yoga, and other fitness videos, viewed a few times then stored at the back of the video collection. Meanwhile, the owners of the stowed fitness equipment and hidden fitness videos sit on the couch watching TV, or most ironically, sit idly on the couch watching athletes work out in professional sports.

There are those few who do work out regularly and faithfully. One of Christie's previous roommates, Beth, would faithfully rise at an ungodly hour every week day morning, jump in her car and drive to the college to swim a mile or so before teaching her 8 A.M. class. Did she take a break on weekends? No. At least one *vigorous* walk each day. And on one notable cross-country ski trip and retreat, Beth managed to effortlessly out-ski everyone else, even the most fit, avid skiers themselves. As even tough, burly guys dropped in exhaustion, they muttered to Christie, "Your roommate is *really* in shape."

Then there's George, who runs religiously five days a week without fail, walks on the weekend, and does calisthenics while watching TV. One would think that after having lived with two such excellent role models for a total of nearly ten years that some of this would have rubbed off on Christie. No such luck.

In Christie's office, you'll find a NordicTrak in excellent condition, covered with dust. There's also a neat little row of free weights in bright, appealing colors. And, somewhere back in the closet, an aerobic video that combines aerobics and free weights. The point is a few of us, a very few of us, manage to make fitness a routine part of life relatively easily. The rest of us have to work at it a whole lot harder.

Most people associate working out with weight loss and focus on that as the primary way to motivate themselves. True, most Americans do need to lose weight; according to statistics published by the National Institute of Diabetes and Digestive and Kidney Diseases (NIDDK 2002), more than 50 percent of U.S. adults are overweight, and nearly 25 percent are obese. As you may know, too many pounds leads to increased heart disease, other cardiovascular diseases, strokes, colon cancer, and diabetes. In fact, so many Americans are overweight that Tommy Thompsen, Secretary of the Department of Health and Human Services, declared that diabetes is now a national "epidemic" affecting some 16 million Americans. That's up 49 percent from 1990 to 2000 (NIDDK 2002).

Sure, some of us are genetically more likely to develop heart conditions or diabetes. Even so, the evidence is overwhelming that healthy eating and proper amounts and types of exercise can change the odds. For example, Christie's dad is genetically predisposed to high cholesterol and heart conditions, but he has always eaten a low-fat diet with plenty of fresh, homegrown vegetables and worked on jobs that required ample physical activity. When he developed a heart condition, he grumbled to his cardiologist that he'd done everything the experts said but developed the heart condition anyway. His cardiologist sharply replied that if he hadn't, he would've been in her office at age thirty-five instead of at sixty. His healthy, lifelong habits had added twenty-five healthy years to his life and had postponed his bypass surgery by thirty years. Not bad.

The point here is, when we live life out of balance, when we fail to get the exercise our bodies need, we develop disease—preventable disease. Many cases today of heart disease, diabetes, and cancer are, in effect, "diseases of choice," as we refer to them. Why diseases of choice? By failing to do what we know we need to do to be healthy, we inadvertently *choose* disease. Yes, many diseases have a hereditary component or are caused by a pathogen (for example, a virus). But our lifestyle can do much to bring on or prevent a great many medical conditions.

So, while working out for weight loss is a good reason to exercise, it shouldn't be the only reason. There are those of us who maintain a healthy weight through healthy eating, but still sit around like couch potatoes.

Maintaining a healthy weight is good, but it doesn't let you off the hook. Muscles need to move, tendons and ligaments need to stretch, blood needs increased circulation, and even the digestive system benefits from increased activity. The human body is simply designed to move, not to sit idle. According to the American Cancer Society, moderate to vigorous exercise is needed to make the proper amounts of, release, and utilize insulin, estrogen, prostaglandins, and other body chemicals (Byers et al. 2002). Cardiologists realize this, of course, and they now require their bypass surgery patients—even those with multiple bypasses—to be up and walking within twenty-four hours of surgery.

In short, a physically active life is a healthy life. Your body isn't designed to remain on idle. The best approach to exercise is to increase the level of activity in the things you already like to do. In other words, take advantage of opportunities to increase your heart rate. If you like music, try dancing around your apartment or house. Or, if you work in an office building, try taking the stairs instead of the elevator. As your body becomes used to extra exercise, not only will your stamina improve, but you'll sleep better and also feel like a million bucks.

The two main obstacles to more activity are, of course, getting started and sticking with it. If you want to make a life change that puts you permanently on the track of better balance and more energy, you have to be honest with yourself and come up with a plan that you know will motivate *you*. For example, Christie finds that if she goes straight back to the NordicTrak after neglecting it, it's much harder and she's less likely to stay with it. What she does instead is routinely walk our two large dogs. This is enjoyable and a good workout. She increases the length of the walks and the frequency, and after she gets back into the routine, it's easier to get on the NordicTrak. Plus, dogs are very good about routine. If Christie neglects a walk, the dogs are sure to tell her about it. The keys here are 1. she makes sure to start out at an appropriate level of exercise so that she feels better after exercise, and 2. she has personal accountability offered *gratis* by her four-foot friends and by the *specific written goals* she's set for herself. For example, she'll write, "I'm going to walk two miles every other day this week" rather than being vague (for example, "It'd be nice if I walked some this week").

A Restful Night's Sleep

Sadly, getting enough sleep isn't always as easy as it sounds. We're frequently amazed at how one of our average days can literally steal away all our energy, both emotionally and physically. And it's after a long, awful day that we especially need to wind down, turn it off, and enjoy a night of undisturbed, restful sleep. But the more exhausted and out of balance we are, the more trouble we often have getting sleep. The stresses of the day can easily keep us tossing, turning, and fretting until the early hours of the morning.

A vital aspect of our program for balance and more energy is your making a concerted effort to get a restful night's sleep. Correcting the imbalances in your life by relaxing can do much to help you find sleep. And as you practice calming yourself and letting go of your daily pressures, you'll find it easier and easier to develop healthy sleep patterns. Just think—no more nights of counting sheep!

Most experts recommend we get at least eight hours of sleep each night, though most of us find it hard to fit that much sleep into our daily schedule. George finds an occasional nap can help. He especially likes to take a twenty-minute "power nap" for a quick boost of energy, especially after lunch.

A few other sleep suggestions are just plain common sense. For instance, don't engage in hard physical activity (for example, aerobic exercise) too close to bedtime. Avoid caffeine drinks and sweets in the evening. Make sure your mattress and pillow are comfortable. And use your bed for sleeping, not watching television or listening to the radio. Simple ideas, but they work!

Sleepless people sometimes look to sedative medications to help them sleep. Most prescription sleep aids are valium-like ("benzodiazepam") drugs or antidepressants, while most over-the-counter sleep aids are antihistamines. Regardless of the type chosen, these medications aren't for use over extended periods of time.

Millions of other adults in the United States prefer to take natural herbal medicines to induce sleep. Three of the most commonly used of these are Valerian, Kava Kava, and St. John's Wort.

Valerian. Valerian is an important remedy in modern herbal practice, given its reputation as an effective sedative. For anxiety-related conditions like insomnia, the root is dried and powdered and given as a tincture or by infusion, often in combination with Scullcap and Mistletoe. Besides aiding sleep, the herb also reportedly tranquilizes without side-effects and is good for headaches, trembling, and other complaints (Gruenwald, Brendler, and Jaenicke 1998).

Kava Kava. Kava Kava has become an increasingly popular herb due to its antianxiety and sedating properties. It's officially approved in several European countries—although not in the United States—for treating nervousness, insomnia, anxiety, stress, and restlessness. Taken to promote sleep and reduce anxiety, Kava Kava's active ingredients are thought to depress central nervous system activity (Gruenwald et al. 1998).

St. John's Wort. Also used to treat burns and skin injuries, St. John's Wort has recently gained a global reputation for its antidepressant and sedative properties. It's frequently used to treat depression, anxiety, and sleep-related problems like insomnia. St. John's Wort is reportedly today's most widely prescribed antidepressant in Germany, and the herb is quickly gaining wide acceptance in the United States (Linde and Bemer 1999). A recent American College of Physicians-American Society of Internal Medicine position paper on treating depression recommended St. John's Wort for short-term management of depression (Gruenwald et al. 1998).

A few words of caution about herbs are in order. Like most anything else taken in excess or over a long period of time, some herbs can prove harmful. Others may cause severe injury. For example, the Food and Drug Administration (FDA) recently began advising consumers of the potential risk of serious liver damage associated with the use of Kava-containing dietary supplements (Center for Food Safety and Applied Nutrition 2002). And because herbal remedies aren't regulated by the FDA, you have to be careful about the quality of the product you purchase for consumption. Even though herbs can be bought at most health food stores, we highly recommend buying them from a reputable, licensed health-care practitioner. At the very least, only purchase brand-name herbals, which usually are more expensive. It's also very common for anxious and insomniac people, without their physicians' knowledge, to use herbal medicines in combination with prescription medicines. Concurrent use of herbs can mimic, magnify, or oppose the effects of either or both. Safety is a major issue with respect to possible chemical interactions when patients use both types of sleep aids simultaneously. Make sure to let your doctor know what you're taking.

Sleep doesn't always come easily or naturally to people. But reducing the negative effects of stress in your life is a great, first step to getting the rest you need and regaining your lost energy.

In Conclusion

The field of health psychology is moving closer and closer to a model of integration that combines the best from both Western and Eastern disciplines. Most holistic lifestyle practices take into account the value of physical, mental, emotional, and spiritual aspects of wellness. Some steps emphasize changing physical conditions through purely psychological interventions, while others emphasize changing conditions through other means. Whatever the particular slant, these models hold that the human body is wonderfully resilient and—with some occasional coaxing and intervening—capable of healing itself. This is why most holistic practitioners work with the "entire person" rather than treat symptoms and diseases. They also stress the importance of self-care and preventing sickness through a variety of methods.

FEATURE:
THE "NEW MEDICINE" AND PAIN

One of the most stressful events any of us can face is unrelenting pain. A pioneer in science-based holistic approaches to the entire person is John Sarno. The author of *Healing Back Pain: The Mind-Body Connection* (1994), Sarno is an attending physician at the Rusk Institute of Rehabilitation Medicine, New York University Medical Center and a professor of Clinical Rehabilitation Medicine at New York University School of Medicine. Since the early 1970s, Dr. Sarno has conducted extensive research into pain syndromes and has identified what he believes to be the cause of most neck, shoulder, limb, and back pain—something he refers to as *tension myositis syndrome* (TMS).

According to Sarno, TMS is a physically harmless condition typified by pain that's caused not by injuries or structural damage, but by a combination of daily life stresses and personality characteristics. His opinion is that, once an actual physical cause of pain has been ruled out, you should look to the psyche as the culprit. As he wrote:

> The idea that pain means injury or damage is deeply ingrained in the American consciousness. Of course, if the pain starts while one is engaged in a physical activity it's difficult not to attribute the pain to the activity. (As we shall see later, that is often deceiving.) But this pervasive concept of the vulnerability of the back, of ease of injury, is nothing less than a medical catastrophe for the American public, which now has an army of semidisabled men and women whose lives are significantly restricted by the fear of doing further damage or bringing on the dreaded pain again. . . . The emotions do not lend themselves to test tube experiments and measurement and so modern medical science has chosen to

ignore them, buttressed by the conviction that emotions have little to do with health and illness anyway. Hence, the majority of practicing physicians do not consider that emotions play a significant role in *causing* physical disorders, though many would acknowledge that they might aggravate a "physically" caused illness. In general, physicians feel uncomfortable in dealing with a problem that is related to the emotions. They tend to make a sharp distinction between "the things of the mind" and "the things of the body," and only feel comfortable with the latter (1–3).

Sarno's approach to the problem of pain is a solid example of the "new medicine" that recognizes the relationship between physical symptoms and emotions, as well as the power of cognitive processing to eliminate many common pain states.

CHAPTER 3

FUEL YOUR BODY WITH HEALTHY FOOD

Eat to live, and not live to eat.

—Benjamin Franklin

Consider these facts from Eric Schlosser's book, *Fast Food Nation: The Dark Side of the All-American Meal* (2002):

> In 1970, Americans spent about $6 billion on fast food; in 2001, they spent more than $110 billion. Americans now spend more money on fast food than on higher education, personal computers, computer software, or new cars. They spend more on fast food than on movies, books, magazines, newspapers, videos, and recorded music—combined. . . . The typical American now consumes approximately three hamburgers and four orders of french fries every week (3, 6).

We're sure we don't need to tell you that fast food isn't good for your health. You already know those burgers and fries have too much fat, which leads to high cholesterol, heart disease, diabetes, colon cancer, and may contribute to other forms of cancer. But how does your diet, especially the consumption of fast food, affect your energy levels?

In the last chapter, we began our discussion of wholesome life-style practices that'll help you rebalance yourself. In this chapter, we address what probably causes most of our woes today—the so-called typical American diet.

Looking for Food in All the Wrong Places

You're tired from a long day at work. It's almost 5 P.M., and you still need to pick up the kids from soccer practice. Earlier this morning, you had every intention of preparing a delicious home-cooked meal for dinner, but now you're having second thoughts. "I'm pooped out. Maybe we'll just stop and pick up some burgers tonight," you tell yourself. "Anyway, the kids love burgers. I'll cook tomorrow." And you swing by the drive-through window of the local burger joint for the umpteenth time this month.

If you know what we're talking about here, please don't feel alone. In our experience, far too many Americans patronize fast-food restaurants. And they do so for the wrong reasons: mainly lack of planning, exhaustion, and being too busy. We even know people who eat out most every lunch and dinner, and we wonder if their kitchens ever get used. Of course, folks who always eat out like this are a dream come true for fast-food restaurant chains. These money-making machines count on your feeling too busy or tired to cook, and they're more than happy to cash in on your lack of meal planning.

Fast Food Means Fast Fat

Let's take a look at the typical fast-food meal. Here's the fat content of America's most popular burgers (according to public domain information from these companies' various Web sites): McDonald's Big Mac, 34 grams; Burger King Whopper, 34 grams; Wendy's Classic Single with Everything, 19 grams. Add to that an order of large fries at McDonald's for 26 grams of fat, Burger King's for 21 grams, and Wendy's for 23 grams. Choosing fast food other than burgers won't help you much: a single medium slice of Pizza Hut Hand Tossed Pepperoni Pizza weighs in at 17.6 grams, a Taco Bell taco has 12 grams of fat (Taco Supreme has 16 grams), and a piece of Kentucky Fried Chicken Original breast contains 24 grams of fat.

According to the USDA Recommended Dietary Allowance, a maximum of 30 percent of calories should come from fat. With the average burger, anywhere from 45 to 55 percent of calories come from fat. In other words, if you consume the recommended 2,000 calories per day, you should eat a *maximum* of 65 grams of fat. The average fast-food meal of burger and fries is 1,100 to 1,200 calories but contains the entire day's maximum fat intake. Keep in mind the numbers we've used here are for the simple burger and fries—no extra cheese, no bacon, no "super-sizing," no milkshake, no dessert.

More importantly, when we're eating foods high in fat, we're not eating foods with other vital nutrients. In other words, not only are we getting too much of the bad stuff, we're not getting nearly enough of the good stuff. Too much fat and too few necessary nutrients. So, with one high fat meal, we've made two strikes against ourselves.

Fat molecules are a rich source of energy for the body. For the body to digest fat, bile from the liver functions like a detergent to dissolve fat in water, helping break large fat molecules into smaller ones. These small molecules that aren't ultimately used up in metabolism are converted back into large fat molecules, which are then transferred for storage in fat cells of the body. This is the main reason why excess calories (those not used by the body) translate into excess fat stores.

Fat is more difficult to digest than carbohydrates. This means fat digestion also takes more bodily energy, which also can zap you. And, of course, we all know what happens when we consume too much fat: it stays with us, and we find ourselves guiltily buying larger sizes of jeans. But the fat does more than just put on the pounds and sit there. By hanging around, the added weight continues to take more energy because, quite simply, carrying extra weight takes more energy. To get a feeling for what we mean, try this experiment: Get a backpack and put a ten- or twenty-pound bag of flour or sugar in it. Put the backpack on and carry it around for a few hours while you do household chores. How much more tired do you get just carrying around that extra weight? In terms of the energy needed to carry that weight, there is no difference between the ten-pound sack of flour and an extra ten pounds of body weight.

Now, you'd think if you're carrying around extra weight it would help you lose weight, right? Sorry. That extra weight makes you more tired, which tempts you to be less active and eat more fats and sugars. This, in turn, puts on more weight, and the vicious cycle hurtles you forward into ever larger sizes of jeans and even less energy. Sound familiar?

Finally, our discussion on fat shouldn't be taken to mean all fats are bad. To the contrary, and it might come as a surprise to you, but there are "good fats" that we need in order to survive and be healthy. These good fats are known as *essential fatty acids* (EFAs), and they're as important to your life and health as minerals and vitamins are. The human body doesn't manufacture EFAs, so they have to be consumed in our diets. The most important sources of EFAs include fish oil, flax-seeds, grape seed oil, and primrose oil (Balch and Balch 2000).

Sugar and Soda

Simple sugars, like *sucrose* (table sugar) and *fructose* (fruit sugar), have a profound effect on your digestive system. In addition to your body needing certain nutrients like vitamins, minerals, enzymes, proteins, hormones, and water, it needs *glucose*, which is the fundamental source of fuel to keep your body going. Without glucose, none of the cellular reactions in your body can occur. But eating more table simple sugars isn't the answer to ensuring your glucose supply. Long-term use of sugar can severely stress your pancreas, which is the gland responsible for regulating blood sugar levels through secretion of insulin. A "yo-yo" effect happens when large amounts of sugar prompt the release of large amounts of insulin. After processing the sugar, the insulin stays around and can then trigger an attack of hypoglycemia (low blood sugar). Consequently, blood sugar levels fluctuate erratically, causing you to eat more sugar, which then prompts more insulin, and so forth. Complex sugars, like those found in pasta, bread, and especially whole grains, don't have this yo-yo effect because they take longer to process.

Put another way, simple sugars crash your system, and you either struggle with less energy or you have to eat even more sugar to get another burst of energy, which will crash you again. The sucrose roller coaster is no way to find balanced energy for life.

Before we tell you how to overcome this potentially depressing pattern, let's look at another part of the typical fast-food meal that often gets overlooked: the carbonated beverage. According to Schlosser, "Americans already drink soda at an annual rate of about fifty-six gallons per person—that's nearly six hundred 12-ounce cans of soda per person" (54). Schlosser has also pointed to the 1999 study from the Center for Science the Public Interest titled "Liquid Candy" that found from 1978 to 1999, consumption of soft drinks by teenage girls doubled and teenage boys now drink five or more cans of soda per day—exactly double the amount of milk they drink.

Have you ever looked at the soft-drink nutrition label to see how much sugar is in a mere 12 ounces? Anywhere from 38 to 48 grams. That's more sugar than you should consume in an *entire day*, and more sugar than is in an average slice of New York-style cheesecake, which averages about 30 grams of sugar. In other words, a 12-ounce can of soda should really been seen as liquid dessert, not a beverage to accompany every meal. And those 32-ounce monster drinks that you find at those gas station quick marts? Those have over *three times* the amount of sugar for an entire day. In other words, one 32-ounce soft drink has as much sugar as the maximum for three days. At that rate you could eat three to four slices of cheesecake and consume less sugar, not that we're suggesting you do so.

"But I drink diet drinks!" you say. Okay, let's look at the carbonation itself. Carbonation contains high levels of phosphorus. Our bodies do need phosphorus, no doubt. This mineral is needed for metabolism, cell growth, kidney function, heart-muscle contraction, and bone and teeth formation—when in proper balance with calcium. The problem is that too much phosphorus depletes the calcium in your system, and lack of calcium, in turn, leads to osteoporosis and brittle bones. The "Liquid Candy" study found that excessive soft-drink consumption led to increased bone fractures in children and teenagers because of calcium deficiencies. Nutritionists have also argued that increased rates of osteoporosis in adults are attributable to increased soft-drink consumption, as well as other factors like too much protein, salt, and caffeine in the diet (Balch and Balch 2000).

With soft drinks and calcium comes a double whammy: if you drink less milk, you get less calcium to start with, and you're replacing milk with soft drinks that deplete calcium. The phosphorus is going to take the calcium from somewhere, and if it isn't in your diet, then it's coming from your bones and teeth. Although it's preferable to limit soft-drink consumption, those who do choose to drink them should be careful to increase calcium intake. Phosphorus and calcium must always be in balance with one another.

But how does calcium deficiency affect energy? Calcium is also a muscle relaxer. Too little calcium can increase muscle tension. Muscle tension can, of course, interfere with sleep and can cause injury when you do try to exercise. The impact of consuming too many soft drinks is tricky, insidious. It can have a dramatically negative impact without our being aware of it because it's indirect and sneaky. We're also less likely to see it as a culprit and may be reluctant to take action against it. We go for the quick pick-me-up and in the process sacrifice long-term, sustained energy.

In addition to the sugar and phosphorus, many soft drinks also contain caffeine, as do coffee and tea. Most people drink caffeinated beverages to wake up or get that morning "boost." But here's the problem with that logic: first, the caffeine shot is temporary; second, caffeine dehydrates. Dehydration, in turn, lowers blood pressure. But isn't lower blood pressure a good thing? In someone with healthy blood pressure, a drop in blood pressure can cause tiredness. So, while that caffeine gave you a kick-start, in the long-run you sacrificed long-term sustained energy for a quickly fading fix. Many people respond by simply drinking more caffeinated drinks, which give another quick boost of energy, but only make the overall problem worse.

At this point in the discussion we ask you to make a choice: now that we've made you really miserable by telling you how much worse your favorite foods are for you than you may have thought, you can choose to give in and be depressed (not our recommendation), or you can choose to be motivated, to take the steps necessary to regain your energy—and your health. When you're making your choice, remember that you don't have to sacrifice the pleasure of great tasting food. We certainly don't.

We know that what we have to share with you works because we do it. We eat well, we enjoy the food we eat, and we stay in balance. Ours is not a quick formula for an instant burst of energy or something you do for a few weeks to "fix" the problem, then go back to life as usual. Our approach is a process of changing little daily habits that gradually add up to a big difference. And the process begins with paying attention to what fuel you're putting in your body and learning if it's the kind of fuel to give you sustained, healthy energy. Eating better means you'll feel better, not just because you'll stand a better chance of achieving your ideal weight, but also because you'll have more energy.

Helping Yourself to Better Nutrition

In order to give the body the fuel it needs, we need to remind ourselves exactly what our body needs and how much. Of course, nutrition is an area of considerable controversy, and it seems new studies of the good and the bad come out weekly. While this may be true, there are still reliable guidelines out there to follow. Keep in mind that these are guidelines. As individuals we may have greater need for certain nutrients than the "average" person; also, men, women, pregnant women, seniors, and children have different needs. If you have specific questions or concerns, you should seek the advice of a registered dietitian and your physician. And you should *never* take excessive amounts of nutritional supplements, as some may become toxic in high doses and/or don't mix well with certain medications.

The best reference is the USDA Food Guide Pyramid, which recommends the following:

Bread, Cereal, Rice, Pasta	6–11 Servings
Vegetables	3–5 Servings
Fruits	2–4 Servings
Meat, Poultry, Fish, Dry Beans, Eggs and Nuts	2–3 Servings
Milk, Yogurt, and Cheese	2–3 Servings
Fats, Oils, and Sweets	*Use Sparingly*

But what is a serving? This is where the advice gets a little tricky. According to the USDA, depending on the food, a serving may be measured in ounces, tablespoons, or cups. Here are some examples from the USDA Web site.

For bread, rice, cereal, or pasta, a serving equals:

- 1 slice of bread (preferably whole grain)
- 1 ounce of ready-to-eat cereal
- ½ cup of cooked cereal, rice, or pasta

For fruit, a serving equals:

- 1 medium apple, banana, orange
- ½ cup chopped, cooked, or canned fruit
- ¾ cup fruit juice

For vegetables, a serving equals:

- 1 cup of raw leafy vegetables
- ½ cup of other vegetables, cooked or chopped raw
- ¾ cup of vegetable juice

For meat, poultry, fish, dry beans, eggs, and nuts, a serving equals:

- 2-3 ounces of cooked, lean meat, poultry, or fish
- ½ cup cooked dry beans, 1 egg, or 2 tablespoons peanut butter count as 1 ounce of lean meat.

For milk, yogurt, and cheese, a serving equals:

- 1 cup milk or yogurt
- 1 ½ ounces natural cheese
- 2 ounces processed cheese

The USDA refuses to put serving amounts on fats, oils, and sweets as it wants to emphasize the message of *Use Sparingly!* (USDA emphasis).

Looking at the recommendations of the food pyramid carefully in comparison to the average American diet, what we find is that, rather than eating according to the food pyramid, most Americans eat something more like an inverted pyramid: mostly fats, sweets, and meat, and not enough fruits and vegetables. To live in balance, we need to get the pyramid back on its solid base of healthy, whole-grain carbohydrates, fruits, and vegetables.

To see what we mean, let's take another close look at the meat and poultry guideline: two to three servings of 2-3 ounces. That's a maximum of 9 ounces for the day. The bottom line is most Americans don't need the large servings of meat they routinely eat. Most deli sandwiches, for example, contain two to three times the amount of meat needed. And most steaks, chicken breasts, and other cuts of meat are double, triple, or quadruple the size they should be.

Overall, most portion sizes at fast-food and other restaurants are much, much too large. Many meals could be cut in half and divided between two people. In fact, when we do go out for dinner, we often ask for the "lunch" portion of the dinner menu item or ask to divide an entrée. Most establishments accommodate this request. Then we can eat reasonable portions without wasting food.

Our Own (Un)Doing

American prosperity has clearly contributed to our penchant for large portions of meat. We have vast land where meat and poultry can be raised, and we have the wealth in our economy to afford the meat. In this way, our prosperity has been our undoing. In other cultures, from Asian to Mediterranean to Indian to South Pacific to South American countries, meat is much more likely to be used as a condiment—that is, chopped in smaller pieces and used in stir fry or other types of dishes. Most often they use far more seasoning with their meats, making them more savory and richly satisfying. The rich seasonings make the meat feel more filling, meaning it takes less to feel full and satisfied. Rarely do you find recipes in these cultures where they serve up a chunk of meat. And in most cases, particularly Asian cultures, they have lower rates of heart disease and other diseases associated with high fat.

We're not saying you should become a vegetarian, though a number of our esteemed—and healthy—friends are. What we are saying is that meat consumption is most often out of balance, and with too much meat, even lean meat, comes too much fat. Look for recipes and ways of preparing meat that are tasty and satisfying, but that use meat in smaller quantities. Here's the trick: if you simply put 3 to 5 ounces of meat on your plate for dinner (assuming you had only 4 to 6 ounces of meat for breakfast and lunch combined), you'll feel deprived. Take that same amount of meat and put it in a beef stir fry, or take that same amount of chicken and put it in a tandoori chicken and vegetable wrap, and you won't feel one bit deprived. We see nothing wrong with the occasional steak dinner, but to be in balance, that should be the exception, not the norm.

We're adamant that the best and first step to a healthier, balanced, and energy-creating diet is menu planning. You know what gets you in trouble: you work hard all day, and you're tired. Everything at home is frozen, or you aren't sure you have all the ingredients to make the healthy entrée you like. Chances are your partner and/or kids have appointments, programs, games, lessons, etc., and you're in a hurry to "grab a bite to eat." You have no idea what to fix and no time to fix it.

The same thing happens at lunch: you're in the middle of a project, you want to stay focused, so you grab the quickest, most available food. In either case, what is available is most likely fast food and most likely high in fat and sugar—those ingredients you now know drain your energy. You grab something quick for take-out on the way home to avoid the hassle and mess of cooking, and have a few minutes to relax in front of the TV. In our modern, hectic lives, fast food and take-out are convenient alternatives when we're tired and stressed. The problem is that this happens at least once a week, and maybe two or more times a week. It doesn't take long for the unhealthy habit to become routine, and it takes even less time to have an impact on your energy levels.

Planning Makes Perfect

To break the cycle and fast-food habit, *you must plan ahead*. And in order to plan, you need to have the resources. Take the money you would spend on fast food and invest in cookbooks that meet your needs. We highly recommend *Cooking Light's 5-Ingredient, 15-Minute Cookbook* (Chappell Cain 1999). All of the recipes take five or so common ingredients and require about fifteen minutes to cook—just like the title says. True to *Cooking Light's* mantra, none of the recipes sacrifice flavor, and they all deliver low-fat, healthy, delicious dinners. A good bookstore, whether brick-and-mortar or online, should have this or similar-type cookbooks geared for the modern, busy, health-aware lifestyle. We also recommend subscribing to a healthy-lifestyle magazine, such as *Cooking Light*. This accomplishes several things: first, you get a monthly reminder and motivation to eat healthy and exercise. Second, you get new ideas and new recipes to keep you out of a rut and motivated. Third, you're reminded that you're not alone in the challenges you face. Fourth, you're challenged to turn off the TV one evening and quietly read the magazine as part of an overall plan of more balanced, energy-creating living!

Once you have these resources, set aside time each week to do menu planning. Now, before you dismiss this recommendation outright, take a look at how we suggest planning. Menu planning need not be a rigid, lock-step, Type-A approach to eating. In fact, if done correctly, menu planning allows for flexibility with less stress. Here's how we do it:

1. *Take a little time to find new recipes that are easy and healthy.* We like to try new recipes regularly to keep from getting in a rut. The more delicious, healthy options we have, the more new things we try and the less likely we are to be tempted by less healthy foods. We look for new ways to prepare and season nourishing foods in healthy ways so we feel indulged at regular meals. This approach takes a little time up front, but the payoff is in less stress later and in better, healthier eating and living, which adds up to more energy.

   To find new recipes, Christie seeks out cookbooks with healthier selections. These days there is a wealth of healthy-cuisine choices, from haute cuisine to every region and ethnicity to down-home comfort foods. Whatever the preferences of your palate, there are healthy options that are reasonable to prepare on a busy schedule. After selecting great cookbooks, Christie then relaxes and reads through them (another activity of more balanced living), looking for recipes she thinks we're likely to enjoy. When she finds one, Christie marks it with a "sticky" tab for later reference. The cookbook shelf in the kitchen now has such a colorful profusion of so many sticky tabs that it looks like a piñata parade! But there is method to the sticky-tab madness, as you'll see.

2. *Select and plan your menus well in advance of your meals.* Either in a chart or list form, write out each day for the next week or so. You might want to make a simple spreadsheet with space to fill in the blanks. Christie uses a basic ruled pad and lists out the days she's planning for. She then goes through the tabbed items in the cookbooks and selects the recipes that fit the week's schedule and fit with whatever might be in the freezer. Because the recipes are already tabbed—both in cookbooks and magazines—she doesn't have to look at every one; she can just go from tab to tab. If she found chickens or Cornish game hen on sale the week before, she goes through the indexes for more recipes with those items.

When she finds a recipe she wants to try that week, she fills it in on the day when it'll work best. Some recipes are more involved and qualify as "weekend recipes," while simpler ones are written in on busier days. She's also careful to select some healthy, family-favorite, old stand-by recipes. Too many new recipes can become stressful themselves, so the mix creates good balance.

Oftentimes, Christie prepares larger recipes on the weekend that'll make good "planned-overs." The planned-overs (not leftovers) make for good lunches or quick dinners during the week on those busiest of days when we're most likely to not cook and give in to less healthy choices.

In all this planning, an absolute rule for weight control and energy management is to *never* skip a meal. That includes breakfast, the most important meal of the day. While we don't specifically plan each breakfast, we make sure there are quick, healthy options in the house: quick oatmeal; lower-sugar, lower-fat cereals; whole-wheat bread, bagels, and/or English muffins; yogurt; fresh fruit; and the like. Skipping meals puts your body into "starvation" mode and causes you to convert more calories to fat. Planning to eat three regular, healthy meals per day is the best way to achieve a healthy weight and gain energy.

Now that Christie has her system down, it takes less than one hour per week to plan delicious, healthy, energy-creating meals for the week. Oftentimes she does her planning while relaxing and watching TV. The time commitment is minute compared to the payoff in health and lifestyle benefits.

3. *Make a shopping list and stick to it while you're in the store.* When Christie has finished planning the week's meals, she quickly

goes through each recipe and makes a list of the ingredients needed. If she's not sure all the ingredients are available or are in season, she may make an either/or list, as in either this or that, depending upon availability. She takes the grocery list and, except for sale items, she buys only what is on the list. Buying sale items and what is on the list, and eating from the grocery store rather than fast-food restaurants not only makes us feel better, it also saves us considerable money.

4. *Carrying out your plan.* This is the easy part because we've already done the thinking and preparation. When we get up Monday morning, something is there for breakfast, and we have something ready to go for lunch. During the day, Christie doesn't have to wonder, "What are we having for dinner?" because everything needed to make a healthy dinner is home in the refrigerator. Either the evening before or that morning she got the meat out of the freezer, if necessary. After a long day of work, she doesn't have to think about it: the recipe, the ingredients, everything is ready to go, and in about fifteen minutes to an hour after getting home, we're eating a healthy, energy-creating dinner. We clean the kitchen together, and we're sitting down to relax by the time our favorite TV shows come on.

Sound too good to be true? We promise, it's not. The key to success is taking that hour or less per week to plan ahead. Think about meals once a week, and then you don't have to think about it again for another week. Once you have experienced the stress reduction of having delicious, healthy food ready, you'll be motivated to do it for another week, and another, and another. Soon you'll have established a new healthy habit, and instead of stopping to pick up fast food by default, you'll go home less stressed because you know what's for dinner and your body is enjoying healthier food.

We'll be honest. Not every week goes perfectly the way it's planned, and, in fact, rarely do we eat every meal exactly the way Christie planned it. Usually we change up a lunch or dinner because we had unexpected or insufficient "planned-overs." Or, maybe something happened and our plans changed. The menu planning makes us better able to deal with the unexpected. First, because we're eating healthier, we're better able to handle the unexpected stresses. Second, because a week's worth of meals are planned, we can switch things around to better fit our schedules. The point is, *it's easier to make changes to a plan than to have no plan at all.*

Another trick to our menu planning: we sometimes plan to eat fast food. What?! Doesn't that go against everything we've been saying? No. Our point is balancing life to attain reasonable energy levels. Never eating fast food is going out of balance in the other direction and puts us at risk to binge on things we shouldn't have too much of. We'll confess we have a weakness for Kentucky Fried Chicken. Once in a while, we simply want it and eat it. With good menu planning, we're then able to balance out the high fat intake. If we have good ol' KFC for lunch, then we have something with no or extremely low fat for dinner, such as salad with fat free raspberry vinaigrette and a vegetable on the side. Light, healthy, low fat, but still delicious. For the overall week, our intake of fat and calories averages out to where it should be. We ate our high-fat KFC and don't have to feel guilty—or tired—for a minute because our overall lifestyle remains in balance.

We also recognize that there are times when fast-food may be the only alternative, such as an informal department or business lunch or when traveling across country. For these occasions, we've made a point of finding out which fast food offerings are the healthier alternatives. In the resources section of this book, you'll find a listing of the web addresses for major fast-food chains. All fast food outlets are required to make nutritional information available, and in most cases the best place to find this is on the Internet.

The best alternatives are Subway's Under 6 Sandwiches, Schlotzsky's Light and Flavorful Sandwiches, and Arby's Light Menu. We've selected these because they're healthy, but most importantly, they taste great. We want to eat in a healthy and balanced way, but there's no way we're going to give up great taste. We like food too much!

If Subway, Schlotzsky's, and Arby's are no where to be found, the next best is a *grilled* chicken sandwich, such as McDonald's Chicken McGrill, which, without mayo, has only 7 grams of fat. But be careful: chicken isn't always the healthiest choice. Depending upon the preparation method, chicken may have more fat than burgers or other menu options. While it's possible to make good, educated guesses in general, many menu items can be tricky for even the most savvy.

We already mentioned that we have a weakness for KFC, and Christie thought she was making a better choice by getting the fresh vegetables in the cole slaw. She knew there was fat in the slaw sauce, but to her horror while researching this book, she found that a single serving of KFC cole slaw has a whopping 13.5 grams of fat and 20 grams of sugar! Servings of the mashed potatoes and gravy, macaroni and cheese, and BBQ baked beans have 6 to 8 grams of fat and are better choices. The best choice, however, is the corn on the cob, with only 3 grams. Likewise, we didn't expect that nearly all of Arby's chicken sandwiches have more fat than their roast beef counterparts, and the "Market Fresh" sandwiches have between 33 and 42 grams of fat—that's more, in some cases, than a fast-food burger! The lesson is this: if you want to make healthier choices, don't assume anything. Ask your local outlet for nutrition information, or look it up on the Internet.

We also feel the need for another word of warning here. No doubt you've seen the ads for Subway with Jared, the college guy who lost 245 pounds eating only Subway's healthy sandwiches. While we applaud Subway's and other chains' healthy offerings and even recommended them here, an extreme approach such as Jared's goes against everything we advocate. Health is achieved through balance. Losing the weight was clearly desirable, but as Maureen Callahan (2002) pointed out in the case of Jared:

> Not only did he skip breakfast every day for a whole year, but he also logged a measly 1,000 calories on each of those days—300 to 500 calories short of the minimum 1,500 calorie mark recommended for most dieters. Missing from his diet: sufficient amounts of nutrients like vitamin E, potassium, and bone-strengthening calcium—all hard to come by when you eat too little. . . . Here's a better idea: make the sandwiches yourself and use the money you'll save to buy a box of high-fiber cereal, a gallon of milk, and plenty of fresh fruit for that missing breakfast (30).

Balance, Balance, Balance

That's right: *balance.* Subway and other healthy sandwiches can be good for a change, but they can't substitute for an overall healthy, planned approach to eating. Once you have a plan and are making healthier choices, there are some other strategies we use to help make food preparation a little easier, quicker, and healthier. If you don't have a pressure cooker, then we strongly recommend you get one and learn how to use it. If your association with a pressure cooker is mushy, overcooked food, then do we have good news for you! Used properly, vegetables come out like they were perfectly steamed. Not only does a pressure cooker greatly reduce cooking times—particularly at altitudes above 3,500 feet—it also retains more nutrients in the food. This is especially true of vegetables, which may lose considerable nutritional value when they're steamed or boiled.

We'd find it far more difficult to practice the menu planning and cooking we preach without the use of a pressure cooker. For most vegetables, we put them in the pressure cooker with some water, put them on the stove on high heat, and bring them barely up to pressure (or use less time for more tender vegetables like asparagus), then quick-release the pressure. This cooks them to a tender crisp state while retaining more of the nutrients. The best part? The whole process takes less than five minutes. Potatoes take a little longer. We can cook potatoes first, keep them warm, then pressure cook the vegetables in less time than it takes to steam the vegetables. Or, one of these days, we'll just get a second pressure cooker.

We've found excellent cookbooks on the market for pressure cookers, which give excellent advice on cooking a range of foods, including dried beans and rice—two food items notoriously slow about cooking.

Many good brands of pressure cookers are available, and you can find independent evaluation of them in *Consumer Reports* and in various cooking magazines. When you purchase one, be sure that parts are readily available after the sale, either through the store where you purchased it or online. Pressure cookers are safe to use if properly maintained (Christie learned to use one when she was five-years-old), but the rubber seal and rubber pressure-release valve must be replaced when they become hard or stretched out. They are very cheap and extremely easy to replace so that even those least mechanically adept need not fear.

If you want to improve your eating habits and attain more balanced energy, make your life easier by getting a pressure cooker as soon as possible. At the other extreme, another indispensable cooking appliance is, of course, a slow cooker. If yours is jammed in the back of a cupboard somewhere, we encourage you to dig it out. Slow cookers somehow manage to be one of the first gifts people give singles and young couples, so we're pretty sure you have one. The problem is, most are underused. Again, many good cookbooks specializing in healthy slow-cooking recipes are available. Find one, and get that slow cooker cooking!

Other Considerations

After trying the strategies in this chapter, you may find that you're still tired. Changing eating patterns won't lead to instant added energy overnight; you'll need to be consistent and give it time. If you do that and still find that you're tired, then you'll need to consider other causes and should seek the counsel of a physician.

If you've recently used antibiotics, they might have killed more than the bad bugs that were making you sick. They may have also killed off the good bacteria that were keeping you well. Bacteria and yeast must maintain a balance in our systems. When bacteria are killed off, too much yeast is allowed to grow, and overgrowth of yeast can lead to tiredness. But as we'll say throughout this book, being tired and exhausted may be the symptom of a more serious illness, and you should seek the advice of your doctor to rule out more serious causes.

If you think you might have a systemic yeast infection, this can be handled with diet and dietary supplements. A reputable health food store with a certified nutritionist can offer some good alternatives, such as the supplement caprylic acid. Grapefruit-seed extract and garlic supplements are also good natural yeast fighters according to Ronald L. Hoffman (1993). These supplements will help reduce the yeast population. Also, most physicians recommend taking acidophilus or tridophilus after a round of antibiotics to restore the flora to your intestines and balance out the yeast. Most importantly, if you suspect yeast may be a problem, reduce or eliminate sugar consumption. Yeast is yeast, and it likes sugar.

You may also want to consult with your physician about the possibility of an iron deficiency, particularly if you're a woman who experiences heavy menstrual cycles. If your doctor determines you're anemic (low in iron), he or she will probably recommend an iron supplement for you. Even if you aren't anemic, you may want to take an iron supplement (pending your doctor's or nutritionist's recommendation). We've found that the most readily available iron supplements on the market are not easily tolerated by some people and cause constipation. You may have to look a little harder, but national chains such as Walgreen's sell good quality ferrous fumerate at a reasonable price that's more easily tolerated.

In general, no matter how well we eat, the experts are now telling us that we may not be able to get all of our nutrients in the desired amount from our diets, though we should get most of our nutrition that way. For example, women of child-bearing age are strongly encouraged to take folic acid supplements. Most people should consider a basic general vitamin supplement. Most women, particularly those at higher risk for osteoporosis, should take a calcium supplement, as most women don't get enough calcium in their diets. People with high cholesterol may want to consult with their doctors about higher doses of niacin.

Fasting

You want to start making healthier, balanced-living choices to have more energy. To this end, we'd also like to suggest that you talk to your health-care practitioner about fasting. Now, fasting isn't for everyone, but most people we talk to tell us how refreshed and rejuvenated they feel after giving their digestive system a little time off.

There are many types of fasts, so you might need to experiment to decide what works best for you. Some people completely abstain from all food and just drink water for anything from a full day to several days. Other people drink only fruit juices. George likes to do a fruit fast once a week (especially after eating KFC!). Some days he eats only watermelon, grapes, or strawberries, and other days he eats different kinds of fruits. Whatever fast you try, the point is to give your system a break—a chance to rest—so that you'll feel more energetic in the long run.

Please, if you decide to try a fast, *you must talk over your plans with your doctor*. Fasting can be hard on first-timers, and you don't want to accidentally aggravate an already-present medical condition.

Drinking Water

We'd also like to remind you to drink lots of water everyday. And we don't mean diet sodas or coffee! Our bodies are mostly comprised of water, meaning you need to drink as much of this elixir of life as possible to keep everything inside you running smoothly. Not drinking enough fluid can lead to dehydration, which can lead to numerous physical symptoms and conditions (for example, headaches, acid indigestion, constipation, dry skin). While some experts now question the need to drink eight 8-ounce glasses everyday, we recommend drinking enough fluids to satisfy your thirst and then some. And if you live in a hot arid climate like we do, it's even more important to drink extra amounts of water.

If you don't like the taste of tap water, you can add a squeeze of fresh lemon or lime. Or invest in a water filter. The extra effort this requires will pay off in a more refreshed, energetic you.

In Conclusion

What we've addressed here are, for the most part, things that are relatively easily remedied. If you address these possible causes and are still tired, this may indicate a more serious problem, and you should definitely seek medical advice and treatment. Tiredness can be symptomatic of serious medical conditions and shouldn't be ignored. Research has found that women in particular are inclined to ignore symptoms of tiredness and exhaustion, shrugging it all off as being busy with work, home responsibilities, and the demands of motherhood. While life's demands can leave you tired, you shouldn't experience excessive, prolonged tiredness or exhaustion.

FEATURE: SNACKS AND MUNCHIES

All the healthy menu planning in the world is useless if you blow it with unhealthy snacking. Oh, we've all done it. We all have our own weaknesses and our own stories. Recently a women shared with us how she couldn't resist that super-sized bag of potato chips in her pantry. She ate the whole bag—and then went out and bought another one so her husband wouldn't know. Then there are those who confess to eating entire bags of Girl Scout cookies, or Chips Ahoy, or . . . the list goes on. Christie has utterly no self control when it comes to anything chocolate mint, particularly chocolate mint melt-aways. She's been known to consume an entire package in one sitting. That blows a month's worth of good behavior!

We all get the munchies, especially while watching TV. In American culture, in fact, TV-watching and eating munchies are strongly associated with one another. To keep ourselves balanced and not undermine the healthy eating we do the rest of the week, we've devised snacking strategies to help us stay in balance without feeling deprived.

First off, it's okay to snack. Yes, that's right. A snack can be good for you if you're feeling tired. George is an infamous snacker; he even calls himself a "grazer" because he prefers lots of little meals (or snacks) during the day rather than three big ones. Why? He finds he has more energy than if he tries to digest huge meals. So, before you run for donuts and chocolate candy bars, keep in mind you have to eat the right kind of snack. Go for low-sugar foods that release their sugar slowly, like bananas.

One of our personal favorite snacks is grapes (especially when we get the munchies at night). They are sweet, and you can kind of munch on them like popcorn. If we're in the mood for even sweeter snacks, dried fruit is a great alternative, especially apricots. Plus, the chewy texture is satisfying. Pretzels are also a good low-fat alternative. We keep fresh fruit in the house at all times. When we want to feel especially indulged, we'll get fake crab and cocktail sauce. This is a zero-fat, healthy snack with the satisfying zing of the cocktail sauce. We can snack on an indulgent treat and stay well within our healthy eating guidelines. If a seafood treat doesn't do it for you, then maybe you would like to try one of these.

Homemade Tortilla Chips
and Bean Dip

Cut flour tortillas into pie-shaped pieces and place them in a 350 degree oven on a cookie sheet or baking stone for seven to ten minutes or until crisp. They may need to be turned when they start to curl after about four or five minutes. Look for vegetarian refried beans at your grocery store. These taste great and they have only 2 grams of fat in a half cup. Heat the vegetarian refried beans in the microwave in a dish with lid (beans explode in a most glorious fashion). Top with some fat-free sour cream and some green onions. Maybe a little salsa. Now you have a delicious, healthy bean dip with healthy tortilla chips without sacrificing flavor. To make it even healthier, try low-fat flour tortillas or whole-wheat tortillas.

Healthy Bean Burrito

Using the same ingredients above, after heating the refried beans, place them in a flour tortilla with low fat cheese, green onion, etc., and you have a healthy burrito. Make smaller ones for a snack or a larger one for lunch or dinner. If making a meal out of it, serve with fresh fruit.

Healthy Chef Salad

Purchase salad-in-a-bag, healthy, low-fat, packaged deli meats, and reduced fat cheese. Put some of the salad on your salad plate and top with slices of the deli meats and cheese. If you haven't already had an egg for the day, add a hard-boiled egg. Serve with a low-fat dressing. You've just turned a salad into a tasty meal or snack that uses meat as a condiment, but doesn't deprive you of flavor.

CHAPTER 4

USE HOLISTIC HEALTH TO LOOK AND FEEL GREAT

Natural forces within us are the true healers of disease.
—Hippocrates

George's work in clinical health psychology eventually piqued his interest in an entirely different area of health care that's collectively known by such phrases as "alternative medicine," "holistic health," "integrative health," "new age health," "complementary medicine," "integral medicine," and "blended medicine." (We prefer the descriptors "complementary" and "integrative," which imply that these methods have a place alongside of—not replacing—mainstream medicine.) The basic idea behind integrative medicine is the goal of achieving general wellness instead of just curing illness. This is accomplished at the multiple levels of body, mind, and spirit. Common holistic tools for wellness include seeking balance, good nutrition, fresh air, physical activity, social interaction, mental stimulation, and time for introspection.

Starting in his mid-to-late twenties, George began suffering from severe migraines and was plagued by them for twelve long years, typically having as many as five major attacks per week. The only approach mainstream doctors knew to take was to prescribe medications, which either had intolerable side effects or limited usefulness in George's case. Eventually, when working as an academic dean and taking courses at the Dallas College of Oriental Medicine, George was exposed to both Chinese and chiropractic methods for treating headaches (as well as a multitude of other conditions). After a few weeks of having cervical and thoracic adjustments and taking the Chinese formulas *Jia Wei Xiao Yao San* and *Tian Ma Wan* (though not at the same time), the headaches were drastically reduced in intensity and frequency. And today, George rarely has migraines, a state that he attributes to his continuing use of adjustments and herbs. Seeing the benefits for George, Christie soon developed a similar interest in the natural approach. She became a supporter when George was able to reduce her tension headaches by pressing specific areas on her back, as well as settle her stomach by rubbing certain areas on her feet.

Given our own personal victories with natural health, we've become particularly intrigued by the fact that *most complementary therapies promote attaining general wellness over correcting disease states.* Although these and other terms might cause some of our mainstream readers to cringe, the fact remains that many forms of health care have existed throughout the world, most of them flourishing long before the development of what is referred to in the West as *allopathic medicine* (mainstream medicine).

Just because a therapy or technique has been around for a long time doesn't make it legitimate. But its longevity doesn't make it obsolete, either. It's possible, for example, that the accumulated knowledge of the last 3,000 years of Oriental medicine has important insights to offer the West with regard to herbal formulas. (Don't forget that many of our standard pharmaceuticals, like their herbal counterparts, are based on plant derivatives.) We believe today's health-care system has much to learn from the practices of the past and from around the globe; American medicine needs to build on the best methods from both West and East. And to do this requires cooperation and mutual respect across disciplines and between practitioners of differing backgrounds, as well as solidly-designed, double-blind, controlled research studies. It won't happen overnight, but we can take some comfort in such developments as the National Institutes of Health having created an Office of Alternative Medicine to research the legitimacy of various complementary methods.

We want to make it clear before proceeding that neither of us presume to be an expert in any of the complementary therapies. Nor do we think a thorough review of three or four thousand years worth of medical history is a practical goal for this chapter. A growing number of lay-oriented books and classes are commercially available that describe and teach nearly every aspect of Western and Eastern models of health care, including mainstream, complementary, psychological, and spiritual perspectives. Instead, we want to give you a very brief introduction to some approaches that might hold promise for sufferers of everyday tiredness. We've found these to be supported by at least some Western scientific research. We also hope that this chapter will show you the value of an *integral model* for overall health care—one that harmonizes care of the body, the mind, and the spirit.

Unfortunately, those who practice alternative health in this country are sometimes apt to criticize Western medicine as disinterested in individual patients, their families, and their social systems. All too often, American holistic practitioners and students bring many conscious and unconscious beliefs about wellness, disease, and healing to their studies. This is to be expected, given the level of media exposure advocating allopathic methods (for example, a medication for everything) that most Americans experience. A majority of these students choose to enter the alternative health field because they favor an integrative approach that's based on more natural healing concepts. This is fine and good as long as these people realize both their strengths and limitations. Additionally, American practitioners and students must be ready to address an interesting dichotomy that exists today. For example, Chinese acupuncturists often argue that TCM should only be practiced in light of modern scientific and technological advances, not in light of mysticism and superstition. On the other hand, American practitioners often argue that the "the ancient ways" must be emphasized, even at the expense of proven Western science. Understandably, none of this sets well with the medical establishment, which often reacts negatively to the entire idea of holistic health. And so the cycle goes.

To reiterate, in our opinion, *there is plenty of room for both allopathic and holistic health professionals who are trained, licensed, and dedicated to work together for the benefit of their patients*. Setting aside the political tangles associated with this topic, let's now consider how four prominent models of complementary health care—Oriental medicine, chiropractic, naturopathy, and massage therapy—might be beneficial adjunctive therapies to the other techniques that we've already described.

Finally, as we mentioned earlier, if you're troubled by physical exhaustion, you do need to see a health-care professional to rule out the presence of a physical disorder. But after you've had all the necessary medical tests, sought a second opinion, and been assured there's nothing seriously wrong with you physically, it's definitely time to begin *rethinking* how you look at life. And if you're so inclined, integrative health care could have valuable benefits to offer you in terms of increasing your energy naturally.

Oriental Medicine

An entirely distinct model of health care is *Oriental medicine*, a complete and coordinated system that's used to diagnose and treat sickness, prevent disease, and improve wellness. Also known as Traditional Chinese Medicine (TCM), Oriental medicine encompasses many diverse Asian health-enhancing and energy-balancing therapies. *Acupuncture* (from the Latin words *acus*, meaning "needle," and *punctura*, meaning "puncture") and Chinese herbology are probably the best-known techniques of Oriental medicine. Other frequently used TCM techniques include *Qigong*, *Gua Sha*, cupping, moxibustion, and *Tuina*—all of which involve ways to manipulate *Qi*—the essential energy of life. Originating in China thousands of years ago, TCM is still practiced throughout the world today, including in the United States.

A Few Basic Principles

To comprehend the inner workings of TCM, it's helpful to understand some of the basics of Chinese philosophy—a thorough description of which is impossible here. The concepts of the *Tao*, *Yin* and *Yang*, the Five Elements, and the Eight Principles are all essential to TCM and its unique role in helping to maintain good health, but can come across as rather intimidating or even strange to the uninitiated reader. Fortunately, you don't need to understand Oriental medical theory to benefit from Oriental medicine.

For the purposes of this discussion, one theory does bear mentioning. The view that we're each governed by the opposing but complementary forces of *Yin* and *Yang* is at the core of Chinese philosophy. This balance of forces is thought to affect the entire universe, including us. Thus, a primary goal of Oriental medicine is to restore the balance between your *Yin* and *Yang* in order to restore health and energy, not to mention prevent diseases from occurring in the first place. Thoroughly understanding such concepts as *Yin* and *Yang* (and many others) allows TCM practitioners to diagnose accurately and treat more effectively.

Oriental medicine, then, looks at health problems like fatigue as an expression of your being "out of balance." That's why in TCM you're encouraged to examine lifestyle, thinking, feelings, habits, and values in order to understand your problem from a larger perspective. Your symptoms (whether physical, mental, or both) are considered to be consequences of ineffective lifestyle habits, as well as your body's striving to restore balance.

The Eastern approach is different from its Western counterpart, in which symptom removal is pursued at all costs. Although the elimination of symptoms is often an important objective in TCM treatment, it's not always the ultimate goal. And because it's your responsibility to preserve your own health and *Qi* balance, patient education is an integral part of Oriental medicine.

The Point: Acupuncture

Even though it's only one of many TCM techniques, acupuncture usually comes to mind when people talk about Oriental medicine. Acupuncture is effective for treating a variety of physical, psychological, and spiritual problems. The procedure originated in China more than 2,500 years ago and has continued to be refined since that time. Although allopathic health-care professionals often express skepticism at acupuncture, its proven potency has been embraced in various parts of the world for millennia. On the topic of Western skepticism, Felix Mann noted in his classic text, *Acupuncture: The Ancient Chinese Art of Healing and How It Works Scientifically* (1973):

> Some doctors or patients may indeed wonder how one can practice a form of medicine where the theories on which that practice is based are possibly suspect. Just as a doctor will prescribe aspirin because he knows what are its effects in the body of a patient, so an acupuncturist will needle a certain acupuncture point because he knows what the consequent reaction of the body will be. It is of secondary importance to the doctor to know just why it is that aspirin has its special effects, no matter how intellectually interesting such knowledge might be. At the time of writing little is understood of why the known effects of aspirin take place, yet aspirin, with its simple chemical formula, is the most commonly used drug in the world (4).

Acupuncture relies on the insertion of fine, sterilized needles into the skin to bring about therapeutic effects. Oriental medicine views health as intimately related to *Qi*, or your life energy. When imbalances in the normal flow of *Qi* within the body occur, disease results. Along with the usual method of puncturing the skin with the fine needles, the practitioners also use heat, pressure, friction, suction, or pulses of electromagnetic energy to stimulate various *acupuncture points* (specific spots on the body that are responsive to needle stimulation).

The goal of acupuncture, then, is to restore health by normalizing the flow of *Qi* through *tonifying* or *sedating* specific acupuncture points. From a Western perspective, this might be explained as varying the electromagnetic fields of the human body. (Acupuncture points have been demonstrated to have certain electrical properties, so that stimulating these points modifies the levels of chemical neurotransmitters in the body.) But whatever its exact mechanism of action, acupuncture seems to work by balancing the movement of energy (including nerve energy) in the body in order to restore health.

Is acupuncture a simple process that can be performed by most anyone? *Absolutely not!* Acupuncturists spend many years mastering Oriental medical theory and learning the finesse required to combine points and perform acupuncture properly. As expert acupuncturist Giovanni Maciocia explained in his comprehensive text, *The Practice of Chinese Medicine* (1994):

> Combining points in a safe, effective, and harmonious way is a very important part of an acupuncture treatment... Using points according to their action brings into play the particular nature of the individual point, while combining points in a harmonious way brings into play the channel system as a whole, and harmonizes Yin and Yang, Top and Bottom, Left and Right, and Front and Back. When points are combined well, the patient has an unmistakable feeling: it may be one of relaxation, elation, alertness, peacefulness or a combination of all these. Ideally, the patient should experience any of the above feelings during and after every treatment (805).

Because acupuncture supports the body's natural healing powers, many conditions can be improved, corrected, or even eliminated. This means the effectiveness of acupuncture extends far beyond the misconception that its only benefit is controlling pain. Acupuncture has repeatedly been shown to improve circulation, lower blood pressure, and increase the production of white and red blood cells. It can reduce gastric acidity and stimulate the immune system, as well as prompt the release of numerous hormones that assist the body's response to injury and stress.

According to data published by the World Health Organization (WHO), acupuncture is helpful for eye and mouth disorders, respiratory and gastrointestinal disorders, and neurological and musculoskeletal disorders. In the United States, acupuncture has historically been used to treat chronic pain conditions like headaches, arthritis, bursitis, injuries, and post-surgical pain. More recently, acupuncture has been used to treat mind-body problems like chronic fatigue, anxiety, stress, insomnia, depression, irritable bowel syndrome, hypertension, sexual dysfunctions, premenstrual symptoms, and menopausal symptoms. Some additional applications of acupuncture include treating drug and alcohol addictions, smoking, and eating disorders. As the National Institutes of Health concluded in its 1997 report on acupuncture:

> One of the advantages of acupuncture is that the incidence of adverse effects is substantially lower than that of many drugs or other accepted medical procedures used for the same conditions. As an example, musculoskeletal conditions, such as fibromyalgia, myofascial pain, and tennis elbow, or epicondylitis, are conditions for which acupuncture may be beneficial. These painful conditions are often treated with, among other things, anti-inflammatory medications (aspirin, ibuprofen, etc.) or with steroid injections. Both medical interventions have a potential for deleterious side effects but are still widely used and are considered acceptable treatments. The evidence supporting these therapies is no better than that for acupuncture.
>
> In addition, ample clinical experience, supported by some research data, suggests that acupuncture may be a reasonable option for a number of clinical conditions. Examples are postoperative pain and myofascial and low back pain. Examples of disorders for which the research evidence is less convincing but for which there are some positive clinical trials include addiction, stroke rehabilitation, carpal tunnel syndrome, osteoarthritis, and headache. Acupuncture treatment for many conditions such as asthma or addiction should be part of a comprehensive management program.
>
> Many other conditions have been treated by acupuncture; the World Health Organization, for example, has listed more than 40 for which the technique may be indicated (online article).

Our point here is that, with the right practitioner using the right techniques, acupuncture might just help you regain some of your lost energy. Many people have found this to be true. But please keep in mind that there are no magic answers. Acupuncture might not help you at all, and it won't be of any use unless you also address your unwholesome lifestyle habits.

We also can't emphasize strongly enough that Oriental medical theory is *complicated*; it can't be learned by reading a book or attending a weekend workshop. It takes many years to become proficient in all of the intricacies of tongue and pulse diagnosis, channel theory, organ theory, and point energetics. Therefore, we advise you to be careful when seeking an acupuncturist or TCM practitioner. Only go to a licensed professional with adequate training in Oriental medicine. (See this chapter's feature on selecting a holistic health practitioner.)

The Healing Power of Green: Chinese Herbs

Like acupuncture, Oriental herbal medicine is a comprehensive healing system that has been refined over thousands of years. It's also used worldwide. For instance, Japanese *Kampo* boasts an updated and proven approach to the ancient art of Oriental herbal medicine. In both America and Asian societies, the most common treatment protocol today involves combining acupuncture with Chinese herbs.

Regardless of the exact approach taken, Oriental herbal practitioners generally develop herbal prescriptions that are carefully tailored to each person's unique bodily constitution, primary symptoms, and chief complaints. In other words, the herbs are used holistically and aren't chosen based only on symptomatic complaints. This is quite a different approach than allopathic physicians take when prescribing drugs, which makes sense given the major philosophical differences between TCM and Western medicine.

According to Oriental medical theory, the human body is a composite of interacting component systems, with each part of the body influencing every other part of the body. TCM herbalists seek a complete description of every patient's overall health constitution and status in order to obtain precise results. In that way, the patient's unique patterns can be identified and the right herbal formula prescribed. Nonspecific allopathic labels like fatigue, headache, influenza, arthritis, ulcer, hepatitis, allergies, insomnia, heart disease, pneumonia, or premenstrual syndrome don't necessarily provide TCM herbalists with enough information.

The bottom line is that the use of Chinese herbs, like acupuncture, requires the expertise of a highly trained clinician. *Never use Chinese herbs except under the supervision of a qualified practitioner.*

Oriental Medicine and Everyday Tiredness

In TCM, the main goal is to correct and prevent imbalance and its consequences—disease, misery, fatigue, and so on. As we noted earlier, ailments of most every type are the consequences of the imbalance (excess or deficiency) of the body's *Qi*, including its *Yin* and *Yang*.

Let's return to our discussion of *Yin* and *Yang*. These terms are used to describe the opposing yet complementing qualities of nature. Here are a few common descriptors of *Yin* and *Yang*:

Yin	*Yang*
Cold	Hot
Wet	Dry
Passive	Active
Stillness	Movement
Quiet	Loud
Slow	Fast
Inside	Outside
Front	Back
Female	Male

See what we mean? Each of these qualities has a corresponding opposite quality. But each also needs the other; for example, it's difficult to understand and describe "passive" without "active."

In an ideal situation, each quality would be in perfect balance with the corresponding quality. But this doesn't really happen, or doesn't last very long if it does. This means life and nature are generally prone to imbalance, and this includes people. The goal of TCM is to restore balance.

Let's take this a step further. Did you ever play on a seesaw as a kid? Remember that excitement when you and your friend balanced each other on the seesaw? Now think of *Yin* on one side of the seesaw and *Yang* on the other. The Oriental medical ideal is for both *Yin* and *Yang* to balance each other. But we know life isn't so simple. Here's what happens. When *Yin* is lower, *Yang* is higher. When *Yang* is lower, *Yin* is higher. Put another way, too little *Yin* gives too much *Yang*, and too little *Yang* gives too much *Yin*. Too much damage to either can be irreparable, even to the point of death. The important point to remember here is the concept of *harmony*.

From the standpoint of TCM, exhaustion (as a form of *Qi* deficiency, discussed under the term *Xu Lao*) can have various causes. However, many cases of fatigue involve damage to the *Yin* from overexerting ourselves. Returning to our seesaw example, lowering the *Yin* will, for a time, result in raising the *Yang*. Ever felt more energetic the busier you become? Sometimes we refer to this as being "wound up" or "running on nervous energy." The reality, of course, is that you can't keep the high pace up for too long. You eventually become depleted and use up your *Qi* as your resources wear down.

When we overdo it, we deprive ourselves physically of regular and healthy meals, exercise, and rest. This, in turn, alters the functions of our internal organs, which disrupts the harmony between our *Yin* and *Yang*, which then brings on tiredness and disease. How? The balance or imbalance between activity and rest directly influences *Qi*. When we're active, we use up *Qi*; when we eat correctly and rest, we restore *Qi*. If you work too many hours or run around like a wild person, you don't have a chance to restore your *Qi* quickly enough. And the result? You use up your essential *Qi*, or your body's primary energy. This drains the vitality from your internal organs, which causes chronic fatigue.

Interestingly, a lack of physical activity can also cause fatigue. This might sound contradictory to the Western mind, but from the Chinese standpoint, a lazy lifestyle can interfere with the free flow of *Qi* as much as a hectic lifestyle. Think of a Saturday morning when you didn't get enough sleep the previous night and felt tired all day. Then consider the Saturday when you slept too much and then felt groggy all day. See how this works? If you get too little sleep, you're tired. If you get too much sleep, you're also tired. Again, *balance, balance, and balance!*

From the perspective of TCM, then, typical causes of damaged *Yin* and depleted *Qi*—with resultant tiredness—include both physical and mental overwork, too much or too little exercise, a long bout with illness, physical trauma, excessive sexual activity, drinking too little water, and malnutrition. The answer is to avoid these, as well as use acupuncture, acupressure, meditation, and other TCM techniques to regain lost *Qi*.

Chinese herbalists might also recommend using tonic herbs for an energy boost. Support Central *Qi* Pills (*Bu Zhong Yi Qi Tang*);

Rehmannia Six (*Liu Wei Di Huang Wan*); and Anemarrhena, Phellodendron, and Rehmannia (*Zhi Bai Di Huang Wan*) are often prescribed to regulate low energy due to a variety of causes.

Oriental medicine is also effective for treating the stress that leads you to feel drained. As one example, an acupuncture point known as *Yin Tang*, which is located between the eyebrows, has a considerable effect on most stress and anxiety reactions. And many Chinese herbal formulas for anxiety contain *Suan Zao Ren* (Semen Zizyphi Spinosae) because of its special calming properties.

In short, Chinese medicine offers an alternative explanation for how problems like everyday tiredness develop, as well as treatment strategies for restoring *Qi*. Depending on your specific clinical presentation, acupuncture and herbal therapy could very well help in your recovery from everyday tiredness.

Chiropractic

The largest and most organized of the alternative therapies in this country, chiropractic is a fast-growing branch of health care devoted to the idea that wellness depends, at least in part, on a normally functioning and healthy nervous system. Derived from the Greek words *cheir* (meaning "hand") and *praxis* (meaning "practice"), "chiropractic" literally translates "treatment by hand."

Doctors of chiropractic believe in the body's inherent wisdom to heal itself, and thus contend that the cause of many dysfunctional processes begins with the body's inability to adapt to its surroundings. Chiropractors look to address dysfunction, pain, and disease not by using medications or surgery, but by locating and correcting musculoskeletal areas of the body that are malfunctioning. This approach normally includes the fine art of spinal adjustments, as well as the use of massage therapy, nutritional modifications, lifestyle recommendations, exercise, and a wide range of other natural methods to promote physical and emotional fitness.

Why spinal adjustments? The human spinal column consists of a series of vertebrae (movable bones) extending from the base of the skull to the pelvis. Thirty-one pairs of spinal nerves continue from the brain down the spine, and these nerves exit through a series of openings between the vertebrae. As the nerves exit the spine, they form a complicated network that affects tissues in your body. Many everyday events can cause these spinal bones to lose their normal positioning. When this happens, a chain of events occurs that influences the spinal cord, nerves, muscles, and soft tissues. When the vertebrae remain out of alignment, the result is an impingement of some of the nerves of your body, leading to diminished functioning. Even small amounts of pressure on nerve roots can reduce the amount or quality of neural transmission to a significant degree, not to mention cause you numbness or pain. Misalignments can also exert tension on your muscles, tendons, and ligaments.

The spinal vertebrae are realigned during a chiropractic adjustment. The result is a release of the impingement of the nerves and stress on your muscles, which then improves overall functioning of your body. As David Chapman-Smith wrote in *The Chiropractic Profession* (2000):

> Accordingly, the goals of chiropractic joint adjustment or manipulation are not only to correct musculoskeletal dysfunction, improving range of motion and reducing pain, but also to restore normal function in the nervous system. This, chiropractors postulate, will improve homeostasis [a state of internal equilibrium or balance of systems] and thus affect body functions generally, improving resistance to disease and producing a feeling of well being. Much of this has yet to be proven convincingly, but it is consistent with modern neurophysiology and explains clinical results in chiropractic practice (60).

The verdict may still be out on exactly how chiropractic works. Many chiropractors speak of correcting the *vertebral subluxation complex* (misaligned vertebrae), while others speak of opening energy channels. Still others speak of restoring the motion of the vertebrae as they move against each other, as very subtle changes in the vertebrae's motion can have a significant effect on the nerves running through them. Whatever the theory held, chiropractic undoubtedly works for millions of people. Yet more research is needed to determine conclusively what underlies the effectiveness of spinal adjustments.

The conditions that chiropractors address are as vast and diverse as the human nervous system itself. For this reason, chiropractors rely on the same basic methods of physical examination, radiographic ("X-ray") examination, laboratory analysis, consultation, and the taking of case histories, just like any other physician. In addition, chiropractors use a standardized, comprehensive chiropractic structural examination, paying close attention to the alignment of the spinal vertebrae in order to diagnose a patient's condition and determine the appropriate course of therapy. This examination to evaluate the structural integrity and function of the spine is the hallmark of chiropractic, making it unique among the various health-care professions.

Chiropractic and Everyday Tiredness

Living in our rigid and high-strung world causes many of us to develop muscular tensions that affect the psyche. This probably explains why so many patients who visit doctors of chiropractic describe stress and anxiety associated with their pain.

For reasons not exactly understood, stress and anxiety frequently strike the weaker areas of the spine, causing pain in the form of headaches, migraines, neck pain, back pain, and general muscular tension. This pain, in turn, ends up aggravating the stress, which then causes more pain. Why? When you have pain, your body and mind are under tremendous stress. You begin fretting, for example, about whether the pain will affect your ability to work, sleep, have sex, and otherwise enjoy life. The stress increases nervous-system activity, which in turns makes your subjective experience of pain feel more intense.

It stands to reason that stress and anxiety are also triggered by fears of anticipated pain (physical or emotional), disease, and death. Chiropractors and psychologists witness this phenomenon daily. That is, *tiredness can result not only from stress, anxiety, and pain itself but also from the anticipation of stress, anxiety, and pain.* For this reason, chiropractic therapy is aimed at alleviating the musculoskeletal conditions that lead to and aggravate both physical *and* mental problems.

You might not initially think of chiropractic as a therapy for chronic tiredness. But if you live a hectic and unbalanced life, you're probably suffering from too much stress. Chiropractic can definitely help you relax. Indeed, much tension, stress, and anxiety are locked within spinal misalignments, which might explain why patients frequently report less stress and more energy following chiropractic adjustments.

The manipulative process of chiropractic also allows you to open up emotionally. When your tension is relieved, psychological issues and memories surface. You then feel more like talking about whatever it is that's bothering you, which is a major first step in making those necessary lifestyle changes we've been describing.

Naturopathy

Naturopathy, also known as *naturopathic medicine*, is the science and art of preventing, curing, and alleviating suffering through the use of treatment methods that are in harmony with the laws of nature. Naturopathic medicine was founded in the United States in the early 1900s by a German physician, Benedict Lust. Later, naturopathy was formalized by such notables as Henry Lindlahr, M.D., whose theories, principles, and recommended therapeutics contributed to contemporary naturopathic philosophy and practice.

This branch of health care combines centuries-old natural techniques with modern medical ones. Naturopathy also draws from the best of healing modalities from many other medical systems, including TCM, chiropractic, homeopathy, and others. The vast majority of today's licensed naturopathic physicians in the United States hold the N.D. (Doctor of Naturopathy) degree and received their training at a naturopathic medical school.

A serious problem, however, for legitimate naturopathic physicians in this country is the availability of unaccredited correspondence, distance education, and online programs that issue (and some might claim, sell) N.D. degrees. The larger medical community has been reluctant to embrace naturopathy, except in several states (for example, Arizona and Oregon) where this form of health care is regulated, requiring practitioners to attend an accredited, four-year residential program and obtain a license to practice. Why? Too many people with these degrees (or even no degree at all) practice as "naturopaths" while cautiously avoiding any semblance of practicing medicine without a license. The political scene with respect to regulating naturopathic medicine does seem to be changing as the lobbying voice in support of regulation continues to build momentum.

Similar to other holistic therapies, naturopathy's focus is caring for the entire person, not body parts or diseases. N.D. physicians treat as wide a range of conditions as other physicians. Therefore, they employ all common diagnostic tools: clinical interviews, laboratory tests, and physical exams.

Treatment, which can consist of everything ranging from vitamin and herbal supplements to saunas and massage, are chosen to work with the patient's "vital force" (basically the same thing as *Qi* in TCM) to bring about natural healing. Six principles of naturopathic healing form the basis of this type of medical practice:

1. The human body's innate power to heal itself

2. Health and disease as influencing the whole person

3. Symptoms not as the cause of disease but as expressions of the body's attempt at healing

4. Avoidance of focusing only on suppressing symptoms

5. Prevention as the ultimate goal of health care

6. The naturopathic doctor as both healer and teacher

Naturopathy is effective for a variety of medical conditions, probably due to this system's holistic approach to health care. Because the focus in naturopathy is on whole-patient wellness—on building health rather than on battling illness—all interventions are tailored to the patient and emphasize self-care and prevention.

Naturopathy and Everyday Tiredness

Naturopathic doctors approach fatigue in much the same way as other complementary practitioners. A wide variety of techniques are available. In addition to taking valerian herbs for stress and ginseng herbs for energy, one of George's naturopathic favorites is *aromatherapy*, in which he smells extracted plant oils to achieve certain effects. Inhaling the aroma of lavender oil for a few seconds does wonders when George is feeling uptight, stressed, and overloaded.

By helping you find physical, mental, and spiritual balance, naturopaths can show you how to reduce stress, rid yourself of negative lifestyle habits, improve your diet, and lighten your attitude—all with an aim of your finding a renewed sense of well being and happiness.

Massage Therapy

As you probably know by now, stress can become a factor in bringing on chronic tiredness. Your goal, then, should be to *manage* the stresses in your life, as it's impossible to completely eliminate them. If you can learn to manage your stress and its effects, you can regain control over both your life and health.

The last few decades have witnessed a tremendous surge of interest in *therapeutic massage,* or the systematic manipulation of soft bodily tissues—in particular, the muscles—for the purpose of relaxing and "normalizing" their functioning to achieve optimum stress reduction and wellness. In other words, a primary goal of massage therapy is to assist the body's ability to heal itself and to increase wellness by decreasing stress, bodily tension, and pain. Massage therapy has been incorporated into many health-care models, including both complementary and allopathic systems. Most massage therapists practice out of their own office, at spas and salons, at shopping malls, or in conjunction with other health-care practitioners, such as chiropractic doctors.

Massage therapy takes many forms, but three of the most common are Swedish massage, deep-tissue massage, and *Tuina* (Chinese pressure point massage). Whatever the style practiced, massage therapists generally utilize any of a number of massage strokes to eliminate muscle tension, including long and broad strokes, movable or fixed pressure, holding, percussion, and vibration. Whereas massage therapists mostly use their hands, some also use their forearms, elbows, feet, or mechanical devices to locate areas of tension and other soft-tissue problems, as well as manipulate soft tissues with the right amount of pressure (based on the client's feedback).

In massage therapy, *human touch* is central to the healing process. Touch conveys a sense of caring, compassion, and empathetic relationship—important ingredients in any form of mind-body healing. According to Frances Tappan's chapter, "The Mind-Body Connection" from her book, *Healing Massage Techniques: Holistic, Classic, and Emerging Methods* (1988):

> The art of healing is a two-way street. A massage given by one who includes the patient as partner will be remarkably more effective than that given as a mere technique of body manipulation. One who devotes total attention by communicating concern, empathy, and a sincere desire to promote the healing process will spur a patient to participate in the effort toward regaining health (35).

What does massage therapy accomplish? From a physiological point of view, products like lactic acid accumulate in overworked muscles, causing stiffness, pain, and even muscle spasm. Massage can assist in the elimination of these and other metabolic waste products. It improves circulation, which increases blood flow and delivers oxygen to bodily tissues, and it probably boosts immune functioning. And it also stimulates release of *endorphins*—the body's own natural pain killers. Blocked, deadened areas are often able to respond to sensory input again. All of these effects of massage therapy can speed healing after injury, enhance recovery from disease, and even prevent illnesses from developing in the first place.

From a psychological point of view, massage reduces stress and anxiety by promoting relaxation. During a massage, your tight muscles relax, and the pain associated with chronic tension is relieved. Massage also enhances self-esteem and promotes a general sense of well being. As a close friend recently told us:

> *I recommend everyone get massages! I've always loved back rubs from my husband. But the first time I went in for a professional work-over . . . well, I can't even begin to tell you how fantastic I felt afterwards. It took me about ten minutes*

into the fifty-minute session to really start to relax. And then I just turned into putty. Massage has changed my life!

Amazingly, we've found our dogs also enjoy massages. All George has to do is use the "M" word, and Chester and Spencer readily submit for this treat. They've even learned how to ask George for a massage! Chester comes up and sits with his back to George, and Spencer gently pats his head on George's side.

Massage and Everyday Tiredness

Massage is probably our favorite means of reducing stress to regain energy and vigor. George has practiced massage since the early 1990s, and believes frequent massages probably do more to improve people's physical, mental, and spiritual health than most any other approach. He'd even like to see insurance companies and other health entities cover massage therapy as a preventative health measure. But that's the topic of another book!

Massage can reverse the damaging physiological effects of stress by helping you to:

- Relax your tense muscles

- Improve your circulation

- Lower your heart rate and blood pressure

- Heighten your personal sense of well being

- Reduce your anxiety levels

As we discuss in chapter 7, relaxation is a very powerful antidote to stress, the most famous of all energy zappers. During relaxation, your nervous and endocrine systems initiate bodily changes that slow your heart rate, lower your blood pressure, improve your circulation and digestion, and relax your muscles—all in counteraction to stress. A great many activities can bring about a relaxation response, including deep breathing meditation, exercise, visualization, or listening to calming music. But, without a doubt, one of the best methods to battle stress and anxiety is therapeutic massage.

Massage won't cure your everyday fatigue, but it might provide some appreciated relief from the symptoms of anxiety, stress, and tension. As well, having regular massages will put you in touch with your body so that you're better able to monitor your body's signals of stress. Then you'll have a clearer idea when your body is telling you it's time to rethink whatever is causing your life to be out of balance.

In this way, massage can play a major role in your recovery from everyday tiredness. By combining massage therapy with the cognitive techniques described in the next two chapters, you can learn to avoid the damaging effects of chronic stress while also taking control of your life and health.

In Conclusion

The field of health psychology is moving closer and closer to a model of integration that combines the best therapies from a broad spectrum of Western and Eastern disciplines. Most complementary practices recognize the value of physical, mental, emotional, and spiritual aspects of wellness. Some therapies emphasize changing physical conditions through purely psychological interventions, while others emphasize changing conditions through other means. Whatever the particular slant, these models hold that the human body is wonderfully resilient and—with some occasional coaxing and intervening—capable of healing itself. This is why most holistic practitioners work with the entire person rather than treat symptoms and diseases. They also stress the importance of self-care and preventing sickness through a variety of methods. The terms *complementary* and *integrative* reflect this unification of the mind, body, and sprit.

FEATURE:
FINDING A HOLISTIC PRACTITIONER

Selecting a qualified complementary health practitioner can be a daunting task. Following are a number of sample questions to consider asking as you screen potential health-care practitioners:

- Are you licensed to practice?
- May I see your license to practice?
- What is your educational background and experience?
- How long have you been in practice?
- What is your predominant philosophy of healing?
- Do you have references I can contact?
- How do you arrive at a diagnosis?
- What does your treatment or therapy involve?

- What are the potential side-effects of your treatment or therapy?

- What are the costs and duration of each treatment?

- Do you accept insurance? If so, which plans? If not, what kinds of financial arrangements are available?

- How long can I expect to be in treatment for my condition?

- How long can I expect to be in treatment before seeing results?

- Are you involved in any kind of teaching, ongoing research, and/or continuing education?

- Are you willing to consult with other health-care practitioners, including medical doctors?

Common sense suggests that you *not* proceed with treatment if your questions aren't answered to your satisfaction. You'll also want to avoid (translate: *run from*) practitioners who:

- Criticize and negate all of allopathic medicine;

- Refuse to coordinate with other health-care professionals;

- Promise cures for incurable diseases;

- Want you to discontinue medications prescribed by your family doctor;

- Pressure you into purchasing expensive herbs, supplements, or devices;

- Require you to disrobe when your "gut" tells you it's inappropriate; and/or

- Make you feel uncomfortable at any time.

PART 2

THE MIND AND EVERYDAY ENERGY

CHAPTER 5

EXAMINE YOUR BELIEFS

The greatest happiness is to know the source of unhappiness.
—Fyodor Dostoyevsky

In this chapter, we explore the theories behind one of the primary causes of everyday tiredness—*cognitive distortions*, or thinking that's based (partially or completely) on untruths, misconceptions, and opinions rather than the way life really is. We'll show you how tiredness is related to unrealistic self-talk and behaviors that prevent your finding simplicity and balance. We'll also give you some helpful tips for a personal *mental makeover*, including how to identify your own misconceptions and overcome exhaustion by transforming your thinking.

The Art of Cognitive Reframing

Undoubtedly, the most effective self-help method for managing everyday tiredness is *cognitive reframing* (or *cognitive behavior therapy,* "CBT," or *cognitive therapy*), which is an area of psychology dealing with why people think and act the way they do. CBT is concerned with the primary role that unrealistic thinking plays in causing you problems. From our point of view, CBT has a lot to offer in terms of improving your life by showing you how to change your thoughts, feelings, and behaviors.

Cognitive therapy is one of the few forms of psychotherapy that's firmly based on scientific evidence from hundreds of clinical trials. Contrary to most other models of therapy, CBT tends to emphasize the present; it helps you figure what you can do *today* to begin overcoming your troubles. This means CBT is oriented toward "here and now" problem solving rather than exploring the past. In fact, much of what you do in cognitive therapy is solve your current problems. You learn specific self-help skills that you can use for the rest of your life.

Cognitive therapy is based on the idea that how you interpret your life affects how you feel emotionally and how you react. For example, you're walking down the street and your best friend walks by but doesn't look your way and says nothing to you. You might either worry that your friend is mad at you, or assume your friend is preoccupied and didn't notice you. In the first case, you automatically assume the worse and fret needlessly, which is irrational. In the second, you draw conclusions based on verifiable information, which is rational. In other words, you have no evidence that your friend is mad, but you do have evidence your friend didn't see you. To draw any further conclusions will only cause you problems. Here we see that it's not a situation that directly influences how you feel or react, instead it's your thoughts—*your interpretation* of the situation.

For whatever reasons—how you were raised, ideas you've picked up from others, the fact you're too stressed—most of us don't always think too clearly. This means your thoughts are prone to be distorted in some way. Cognitive reframing helps you recognize your unrealistic thoughts by learning how to evaluate them. You can then learn how to change these irrational thoughts into rational ones. (Remember, our use of "irrational" simply implies "unrealistic." It isn't meant to be an insult in any way.) And when you think more rationally, you feel better and make life decisions that are in your best interest. With enough practice, your new cognitive skills will become second nature, and your experience of stress, imbalance, and exhaustion will begin to fade away.

In this way, cognitive reframing is an active, educational approach to self-help. But CBT isn't some sort of magic answer to all your troubles. To benefit from CBT, you have to spend time mastering the techniques. Put another way, you've got to *practice, practice, practice.*

The more effort you put into changing your life, the more rewards you'll reap.

Cognitive reframing involves three basic steps:

1. Identifying your distorted ideas

2. Challenging your distorted ideas

3. Rethinking away your distorted ideas

Superficially, this might sound easy, but cognitive reframing takes time and effort on your part. Of course, your problems didn't develop overnight; why expect them to go away easily and quickly? Let's look a little closer at how thinking affects life in general, and then see how CBT principles apply to overcoming everyday tiredness.

Essentials of Cognitive Reframing

According to the principles of CBT, beliefs, life events, emotional reactions, and behaviors all interact and affect one another. Of special importance is the direct influence that beliefs (thoughts, evaluations, attitudes) have on emotions and behaviors. From the perspective of this "Event-Belief-Reaction" model, it's your *interpretations* of people and circumstances that prompt you to feel and act the way you do—not the people or circumstances themselves. For example, the woman who continually tells herself that she can't say no when asked for favors might overcommit herself to the point of developing overwhelming stress, exhaustion, and even physical illness. She might beat up on herself and feel like a failure for being such a pushover. The more this woman engages in negative thinking, the more she believes and tells herself she's a doormat, gets depressed about it, feels more physical discomforts of stress, and so forth—all of which reinforce and perpetuate a menacing cycle of disappointment, self-pity, self-defeat, increased physical symptoms, and chronic tiredness.

Most of the time when you're upset, you're convincing yourself that something is *awful* or *terrible* rather than merely *inconvenient*. Psychologists refer to this process as *awfulizing* or *catastrophizing*. Put another way, if you're a catastrophizer, you might decide that your not keeping a hyperactive schedule is *dreadful* because people will think you're lazy. Or, you might conclude people think your parenting skills are a *disaster* if you don't run your kids to umpteen activities every afternoon or buy them everything they want.

Whenever you believe something in life is *horrible* or *disastrous* instead of merely *unfortunate* or *unpleasant*, you've probably drawn a number of false conclusions, like these:

- The situation, which is totally bad, makes me utterly miserable.

- The condition shouldn't exist because I don't like it. I can't tolerate the predicament for one minute longer.

- I have to find a perfect solution to and fix the situation, or else I'm a defective person and a human dud.

You might also keep in mind that the vast majority of our daily problems, hassles, and disappointments come from *demanding* rather than *preferring* types of thinking. When you feel angry, anxious, nervous, irritated, or guilty, you don't just desire or prefer something, you *require, demand,* and *dictate* that you get what you want. As a case in point, a woman might *demand* that she lose weight quickly and easily, and then become *hostile* when it doesn't happen. Or, she might *expect* that exercise will be effortless and fun, and *browbeat* herself when she figures out it's hard work.

For people with everyday tiredness, these and many other irrationalities are common. This is why research has consistently shown that cognitive reframing can successfully reduce tiredness and restore balance by:

- Teaching you to redefine your experience of everyday life and accept a simpler life

- Helping you to develop active coping strategies (for example, relaxation procedures for those times when you're overly stressed)

- Teaching you a new way of looking at yourself and your lifestyle habits

Types of Distorted Beliefs

Generally speaking, people engage in many types of irrational thinking. If you're preoccupied with avoiding rejection or working too hard, you can probably relate to this. For instance, maybe you've had thoughts like:

- I have to know with complete certainty that everyone accepts me.

- If I don't keep up a sixty-hour work week, my boss and coworkers will think I'm not carrying my share of the load.

- It's terrible if people think I'm slow moving.

- I must be busy (or at least look busy) all the time.

- I can't enjoy free time.

- To be faithful to my religion, I need to volunteer my every spare waking hour at my house of worship.

- My kids will only love me if I give them 120 percent.

- Bigger and newer is always better.

These and a myriad of other distorted beliefs are known by many names, including *irrational beliefs, cognitive distortions, crazy-makers, nonsensical notions, toxic ideas, negative automatic thoughts, negative self-talk,* and so on, depending on the clinician or author. Whatever term is used, cognitive distortions of every type share a common theme: they block your goals and usually fail the test of reason. For example, the belief, "I must be appreciated" fails the test of logic, as there is no guarantee that you'll always be appreciated, and there is no evidence that you really *must* be appreciated just because you want to be. It's nice when people appreciate us, but it's hardly an absolute necessity for survival.

Unreasonable beliefs also lead to more stress and anxiety that block your ability to take it easy and enjoy life. They also lead to such negative emotions as depression, anger, guilt, and shame, as well as such destructive behaviors as workaholism, social withdrawal, hostility, alcohol abuse, and other self-defeating behaviors. As one friend confided to us:

> I keep pushing myself harder and harder. Most of the time, I'm not even sure why. I guess I was programmed as a kid to be an overachiever—to try to be everything to everyone. Anyway, as I've gotten a little older, it's all started catching up with me. I used to be able to work all hours of the day and night and not think much about it. But years of overdoing it have begun to take a toll on me. These days I'm stressed, worn-out, and feel like reaching for the bottle to help me keep going.

Reasonable beliefs, on the other hand, help you reach goals and are sound in terms of logic and reason. They lead to such positive emotions as enthusiasm, excitement, curiosity, joy, happiness, as well as such constructive behaviors as slowing down, reflecting on life, tackling unpleasant but necessary chores, facing inevitable conflicts, and risking possible rejection.

In his book, *How to Stubbornly Refuse to Make Yourself Miserable About Anything, Yes Anything!* (1988), psychologist Albert Ellis proposed that all cognitive distortions are based on three absolute *musts*:

- **Must #1:** I *must* perform well and/or win the approval of important people, or else I'm an inadequate person! (demands about self)

- **Must #2:** You *must* treat me fairly and considerately and not unduly frustrate me, or else you're a rotten individual! (demands about others)

- **Must #3:** My life conditions *must* give me the things I want and have to have in order to keep me from harm, or else life is unbearable and I can't be happy at all! (demands about the world)

And here are some additional categories of distorted beliefs collected from the writings of other psychological experts, including Aaron Beck (1979), Arnold Lazarus (1993), and David Burns (1999):

- *Accusing*: Blaming others without the necessary evidence

- *All-or-nothing thinking*: Seeing your life in "black-or-white" terms

- *Damnation* (negativizing): Being excessively critical of yourself, others, and the world

- *Emotional reasoning*: Assuming your emotional state reflects the way things really are

- *I-Can't-Take-It-Another-Minute-itis* (very low frustration tolerance): Easily becoming frustrated when your wants aren't met

- *Jumping to conclusions*: Drawing conclusions about people and events without the necessary evidence

- *Magnifying* (emphasizing the negative, catastrophizing): Overstating the negative aspects of a situation

- *Mental filtering*: Focusing on specific details at the expense of other important details within a situation

- *Mind reading* (fortune telling): Presuming to know what others think, feel, or plan to do

- *Minimizing* (downplaying the positive): De-emphasizing your positive characteristics and accomplishments

- *Overgeneralizing*: Using words like *never* and *always*; applying the characteristics of one member to an entire group

- *Perfectionism*: Requiring that everyone and everything in the universe be flawless and without blemish

- *Personalizing*: Blaming yourself for some negative event

People engage in these kinds of irrationalities all of the time. Just listen to others—and to yourself—and you'll see just what we mean.

Nonsensical thinking can also take the form of numerous *cognitive blocks* that interfere with healthy and intelligent living. Cognitive blocks often begin with words like, "What if. . . ?" "I can't. . . !" "How awful. . . !" or "Oh no. . . !" Here are a few possible cognitive blocks of overly stressed, exhausted people:

- What if I don't make enough money this year?!

- I can't ever slow down!

- How awful it'd be if I couldn't eat fast food!

- Oh no, it's time to exercise again!

Now, let's take a closer look at the particular perspective of the most famous proponent of CBT, psychologist Albert Ellis.

Albert Ellis' Rational-Emotive-Behavior Therapy

Ellis' particular slant on CBT is known as *rational-emotive-behavior therapy* (REBT). Don't let the long string of words throw you. The approach is straightforward. According to Ellis, REBT is an action-oriented approach to emotional growth that stresses your capacity for creating, altering, and controlling your emotions. REBT places a great deal of emphasis on the "here and now," that is, on your current attitudes, painful emotions, and ineffective behaviors that can sabotage your happiness. Ellis believes in teaching people how to overcome the past by focusing on the present, as well as how to make effective changes in life.

Ellis labels behaviors that are self-defeating as *irrational*, and behaviors that are self-helping as *rational*. If you have problems, Ellis recommends you become "more rational." In this way, you can increase your effectiveness and happiness at work, at home, at school, or just about anywhere else.

Like the CBT methods described in the previous section, Ellis proposes that emotional reactions aren't directly caused by events, but by one's beliefs about those events. In particular, Ellis uses an "A-B-C" model to describe the process of identifying and challenging irrational beliefs. In this theory, A stands for *activating event*, which is an external event or situation of some sort that has prompted irrationality. Here B represents *belief*, C represents *upsetting emotional consequence*, D represents *dispute*, and E represents *new emotional consequence* or *effect*.

To illustrate, let's take the example of a person who's afraid to ask for a raise. Marcel has worked for company XYZ for several years, and he's due for some kind of salary increase. According to REBT, A refers to the situation of anticipating a "money matters" chat with his boss, while C refers both to the nervousness from thinking about asking for money and to the avoidance of what Marcel fears. REBT holds that it isn't A that directly causes C, but rather the B (the belief or beliefs) that Marcel has about A. Moreover, A influences B in the sense that without needing extra money or feeling deep-down that he deserves a raise, Marcel's distorted beliefs are less likely to occur. B influences A in that whether Marcel approaches A is influenced by his beliefs regarding both the appropriateness of asking for a raise and his willingness to do so. C influences B in that Marcel's feelings affect the likelihood of his having distorted thoughts.

So, the more nervous Marcel is about talking about money with his boss, the more likely he is:

- To worry about his nervousness being seen by coworkers and others around him

- To expect a negative response from his boss

In a similar way, C influences A because when Marcel is anxious, he might also be more likely to avoid the A of asking for a raise, even if it's necessary to do so. Finally, A can directly influence C, as, for example, when Marcel receives an undesirable reaction, such as his boss becoming angry or insulted.

We can outline Marcel's situation according to Ellis' A-B-C model this way:

A. *Activating event*: Anticipating having to ask the boss for a raise at an upcoming performance review

B. *Beliefs*:
   - I know I'll freeze up and not be able to ask him for more money. (overgeneralizing)
   - What if my boss gets mad and fires me on the spot? That'll be really terrible. (catastrophizing)
   - If I freeze up, I won't be able to stand it. It'd be awful (catastrophizing), and I'd be less of a person. (self-berating)

C. *Consequences* (emotions and behaviors):
   - Lots of stress and anxiety symptoms

- Extreme everyday tiredness
- More physical symptoms (for example, headaches, sweaty palms, ulcer pain)
- Freezing up or avoiding asking the boss for a raise
- Feeling like a failure for not asking

D. *Disputes* (rational challenges)
- How do I know that I'll freeze up? Maybe I will, but hopefully I won't, particularly if I work very hard at challenging my irrational beliefs.
- It might be possible I could get fired, but it's not very likely.
- If I did freeze up, I could stand it, even though I wouldn't like it. It'd be unfortunate but not really catastrophic.
- How is my worth as a person determined by my ability to ask for a raise? It isn't! At worst, it's a problem for me, but I'm not the same as my behaviors!

In short, while REBT admits a relationship among situations, thoughts, feelings, and behaviors, at the core of Ellis' model is the idea that *beliefs play a primary role in creating and maintaining emotional disturbance, including everyday tiredness.* By recognizing your behavior and transforming your thinking, you can give yourself that liberating mental makeover.

Following are a few more REBT ideas that can influence self-help therapy for the stresses, irritations, and unhealthy thoughts that keep you from eliminating stress and feeling better.

Disturbance and Discomfort

Ellis proposes two essential forms of emotional upsets that are consequences of holding onto irrational *musts* (for example, "I must get what I want"): ego disturbance and discomfort anxiety.

Ego disturbance refers to anxiety, depression, and other emotions and behaviors that result from rating yourself as inadequate, inferior, or worthless if you don't perform certain tasks well or if you fail to obtain desired love or approval from others. *Discomfort disturbance* refers to anxiety, depression, and other emotions and behaviors that result when your demands for comfort or the absence of discomfort aren't met.

Everyday tiredness occurs when those pesky *musts* keep you from making the choices you need to find peace, simplicity, and balance. If you feel worthless to help yourself overcome life's complications, you're experiencing ego disturbance. If you feel angry or depressed at having hassles in life, you're experiencing discomfort disturbance.

Self-Acceptance

For practical reasons, REBT promotes self-acceptance rather than self-esteem. According to Ellis, *self-esteem* involves self-rating (for example, "I'm a good person when I feel good well, display positive characteristics, or get what I want. I'm less of a person when I feel lousy, display negative characteristics, or fail to get what I want"). *Self-acceptance* involves receiving yourself as you are today.

REBT urges self-acceptance rather than self-rating for several reasons. First, human beings are "in-process" and constantly changing. Second, there's no accurate way to measure human characteristics. Third, it's impossible to keep track of all personality characteristics and behaviors. If you rate yourself as weak or inferior because you're feeling burned out, you're on the road to overgeneralizing.

Anti-Catastrophizing

Ultimately, you learn from REBT that most things in life aren't truly catastrophic—that is, absolutely bad. Many stressors, like bad health, are plainly unfortunate and undesirable, but none of them is truly awful, horrible, or catastrophic. You need to accept this tenet of REBT if any of the other described techniques or philosophical ideas are to prove beneficial.

De-Stressing

A number of REBT methods lead to reducing stress. This includes helping you not only *feel* much better and get over some of your anxieties, but also make yourself less prone to becoming disturbed over daily matters. With practice, you should rarely become seriously distressed about *anything*.

Higher Frustration Tolerance

Ellis also instructs his clients in how to raise their frustration tolerance. In this way, you convince yourself that you usually don't *need* what you *want*, that you can stand losses and rejections, and that frustration may be vexatious and aggravating, but that it's never awful, horrible, or catastrophic.

Unconditional Positive Regard

Also important to peace of mind is *unconditional positive regard*, or the ability to accept others no matter what they do or how they act or fail. This means that you accept the essential goodness and integrity of others and yourself, even if their (or your) *behavior* is less than perfect. By always avoiding rating yourself or others, and instead rating deeds, traits, and acts, you can learn patience.

Real-Life Practice

Ellis generally recommends real-life, activity-oriented practice, often referred to as "homework assignments," to help you improve your ability to handle difficult situations. You're encouraged to stay with or endure frustrating situations so that you can learn to tolerate unpleasantness.

FEATURE:

PERFECTIONISM AND CRITICISM

Any explanation of cognitive distortions would be incomplete without a mention of the personality trait of *perfectionism*, which is the irrational pursuit of orderliness, exactness, precision, flawlessness, faultlessness, and impeccability. As Martin Antony and Richard Swinson explained in their book, *When Perfect Isn't Good Enough: Strategies for Coping with Perfectionism* (1998):

> Perfectionism is a problem when it leads to unhappiness or interferes with functioning. Having excessively high standards can affect almost any area of life, including health, diet, work, relationships, and interests (27).

Central to the trait of perfectionism is an *obsessive worry* about controlling everything in life—an impossible task that eventually leads to chronic tiredness and burnout. From the perspective of Allan Mallinger's and Jeannette DeWyze's book, *Too Perfect: When Being in Control Gets Out of Control* (1992), perfectionists and obsessives share a common desire for overcontrol:

Everyone needs some self-control, and some mastery over his or her environment, just to survive. But many obsessives have a *disproportionate* need for control—one that is driven and rigid, rather than reasonable and flexible.

This exaggerated need stems from an irrational conviction that perfect control can ensure safe passage through life. In my opinion, every obsessive person subscribes to the myth that ultimate control is possible, though in almost every case he or she is unaware of it. Like some deeply buried tree root, the "Myth of Control" anchors and constantly nourishes the controlled and controlling behavior so familiar to anyone close to the strongly obsessive person (14).

In other words, if you're a perfectionist, you probably obsess over needing to control other people and your surroundings. Of course, this is a futile attempt. Hopefully by now you realize that *you can't truly control anyone or anything else; you can only control the way you see things, feel, and react.* When you try to do otherwise, you end up frustrated and stressed. And if you keep it up for long, you'll burn yourself out.

Another personality trait that can wear you down is oversensitivity to criticism. That is, we've noticed a tendency for people with chronic tiredness to be unusually sensitive to other people's criticism. No one truly enjoys criticism, especially when it seems that the other person's intent is to hurt or manipulate. But like so many of the potential negatives we've described in *Stop Feeling Tired!*, it's not the intent or nature of the criticism that makes the difference—it's how you interpret and accept it. In other words, you can look at criticism as a threat to your self-esteem, or you can consider the source, forget about it, and go on about your business. It might be *unpleasant* when a spouse accuses you of being a bad parent, but it's not *awful*. You don't *have* to believe what they say. They might think you're lazy, but there's no golden rule that requires you to see things the same way they do.

The ability to handle criticism without "losing it" is a useful skill to add to your repertoire of psychological strategies. But before going any further, we think it's helpful to distinguish between two types of criticism: *constructive* (friendly) and *destructive* (unfriendly). The first is meant to be helpful, is normally delivered by someone who cares about you and your feelings, and is generally welcome; the second is hurtful, delivered by someone who doesn't care, and is never welcome. Constructive criticism can be quite valuable: its main intent is to help you learn a thing or two about yourself, develop as an individual, or enhance your performance in a particular area. Destructive criticism is neither valuable nor helpful: its main intent is to malign, belittle, and control you. When people think of "criticism," they tend to conjure up the negative images and feelings associated with the destructive type.

Dealing effectively with either type of criticism involves knowing what to think, say, and do. One of the first questions you want to ask yourself when criticized is, "Is this person's criticism valid?" Many times people give each other constructive criticism because they care about and want to help each other. There's always the possibility that a particular criticism could be true. Then again, people are imperfect and sometimes offer one another erroneous criticism. Only *you* can decide what you'll accept as true and what you won't. In the end, regardless of the content of the criticism, it's always important to remember that we're entitled to our own opinion.

At the heart of many exhausted people's oversensitivity to criticism lie several *musts* of perfection, approval, and duty. Learning to tolerate criticism, then, involves rigorously disputing and challenging your cognitive distortions of *demandingness*. Three very typical irrational beliefs related to oversensitivity to criticism are:

1. I *must* be absolutely perfect in every respect; otherwise, I'm a bad person, and no one will love me.

2. Others *must* accept and approve of me in every respect, otherwise I'm not a good person, and life isn't worth living.

3. I *must* only hear what I want to hear, as I can't tolerate the discomfort of listening to someone tell me about my faults.

It's also helpful not to take criticism personally, which is what most of us tend to do. Typically, the person making criticisms is actually making remarks about something you're *doing*, not about who you are as an individual. The trouble begins when you *personalize* criticism—when you apply what the other person says about your behavior to your self-worth. If you're ever tempted to do this, just remember that *you aren't what other people say or think.* Just because someone claims you're a lazy bum doesn't mean that you actually are. Why believe you're a bad person just because someone else says so? Stick to the facts, and ignore the rest of it.

CHAPTER 6

TRY A NEW POINT
OF VIEW

It is the mind that maketh good or ill,
that maketh wretch or happy, rich or poor.

—Edmund Spenser

Now that we've learned about one of the primary influences on chronic tiredness—cognitive distortions—let's see exactly what you can do to reduce the stresses and aggravations that cause you to be tired all the time. In this chapter, you'll learn how to dispute your unrealistic thoughts, replace them with realistic thoughts and self-talk, and stop destructive thinking before it ever starts.

Obviously, if you suffer from everyday tiredness, your goals are:

- To become more reasonable about your limitations

- To eliminate excessive stress by simplifying your life and changing your lifestyle

- To find peace within yourself

This is where cognitive reframing can be helpful. CBT gives you a way to look for those distorted beliefs that are suspected of keeping you miserable. And when you challenge your negativities, you're committing to being as rational as possible.

We do want to warn you against engaging in "overly positive" thinking. While "warm and fuzzy" can feel really good in the short-run, false positive thinking is an irrationality in its own right. Consider what the authors of *The 60-Second Shrink: 101 Strategies For Staying Sane in a Crazy World* (1997), Arnold Lazarus and Clifford Lazarus had to say on this topic:

> But there is a big difference between healthy optimism and the Pollyanna pop psychology version of positive thinking. Giddy positivism advises us to look on the bright side at all times. These trite pep talks often tend to backfire and cause resentment and isolation in others.
>
> People who play the "everything-will-be-terrific" game not only overlook real problems and issues that need to be addressed, but they prevent others from expressing grief, pain, anger, loneliness, or fears. It is difficult if not impossible to air your true feelings in the presence of one of these ever-positive thinkers. They often make others feel guilty for harboring bad feelings (31).

Put another way, fooling yourself into a false sense of positive thinking isn't rationality. It's its own cognitive distortion!

Having identified some of the primary causes of emotional distress, as well as having decided not to fall into the trap of Pollyanna positivism, let's now consider the means of reinterpreting life's problems by modifying our thoughts.

Challenging Your Cognitive Distortions

First, to overcome your nonsensical thinking, you accept the fact that you're a fallible human being (or "FHB"). By embracing your humanity, you lay the foundation for overcoming your energy-zapping concerns about looking busy, pleasing everyone, or needing the latest model of this or that gadget.

Second, you quit *demanding* and *complaining* about not getting what you want when you want it. You let go of the *shoulds*, *oughts*, *musts*, and *needs*. Only then will you enjoy a more realistic attitude of *accepting* and *preferring*.

Third, you take away the terribleness and horribleness from whatever aspects of life bother you, and acknowledge that almost nothing in life is, in fact, ever more than *unfortunate* or *inconvenient*.

Finally, you admit that problems, conflicts, stresses, and upsets are, in fact, opportunities for personal growth, not defeat! In other words, you take control of your thinking and *you decide that you can reframe virtually anything so that you can move forward and rationally address it.*

As mentioned above, this entire process of challenging and eliminating irrationalities involves three essential steps. The first step involves *identifying* and *considering* your irrational or unhealthy beliefs, while the second involves *disputing* and *challenging* these beliefs, after which you *replace* them with new, rational beliefs. Disputes often look like this:

- Where is the rule that says. . . ?

- What proof do I have that. . . ?

- Who says. . . ?

- Who cares if. . . ?

- What is the probability that. . . ?

- What is the worst thing that would happen if. . . ?

- Why do I need to. . . ?

- So what if. . . ?

American society has certainly provided us with loads and loads of opportunities to overdo it. If you've ever been on such a tight schedule that it seems like you don't even have time to go the bathroom, then you know what we mean.

Choosing to work too hard can be a major cause of tiredness. Here are some cognitive distortions and disputes for a typical workaholic who can't sleep at night, even though she's "dead tired":

- Nothing must interfere with my work, because that'll be disastrous. I'll lose my job, and I'll feel miserable and hate life forever.

- I must be able to fall asleep easily whenever and wherever I wish no matter how stressed I feel; otherwise, tomorrow will be unbearable, and I can't be happy at all.

- It's horrible if I don't get my work done quickly and effortlessly. Nothing must get in my way!

- If I don't accomplish everything I want to, then I'm automatically inadequate and worthless.

And now for some sample disputes and sensible answers to these irrationalities:

- Where is the law that says nothing must interfere with my work? Why is it necessarily disastrous if a project takes another day or two?

- It's inconvenient if I can't get what I want or can't fall asleep when I'm stressed out, but it certainly isn't terrible. I can stand it. Maybe my best bet is to choose to cut out some of my stress, and then I'll sleep better.

- Sometimes life stinks and things get in my way! But there's no reason for me to get upset about it. Tomorrow always brings new opportunities.

- My self-worth isn't dependent at all on my accomplishments. It might be nice when I can clear my desk, but I'm certainly not inadequate or worthless if I can't.

See how this works? Let's try a few more reframes. To get rid of those nonsensical ideas involving your *having* to stay busy, or the *terribleness* of losing your self-respect if you can't find freedom from life's problems:

1. Identify your *distorted beliefs*, such as:
   - I *must* keep busy at all times.
   - I *must* have the latest and fastest computer equipment.
   - I *must* always be 100 percent in control of everything.

2. Consider how your demanding *musts* inevitably lead to *catastrophizing*:
   - If I don't keep busy at all times, people will think I'm lazy, and that would be horrible.
   - If I don't have the latest and fastest computer, that would be unbearable.
   - If I'm not always 100 percent in control of everything, then I'm a bad person, or I'll look an idiot.
   - If life is horrible and I'm a failure and a worthless person, then I won't be able to stand it.

3. Devise *disputes* that challenge your irrational thinking:
   - So what if people think I'm lazy? What's so horrible about that?

- If I don't own the latest computer, why is that so unbearable?
- Where is the proof that if I'm not always 100 percent in control of everything, then I'm a goof?

4. Finally, create *sensible replies* that answer your disputes:
   - It's inconvenient and undesirable if people think I'm lazy, but it isn't horrible.
   - It's uncomfortable when I don't get everything I want, but that doesn't mean I can't bear it.
   - It's unrealistic to think I can control everything. When I can't, there's absolutely no proof that I'm a goof as a person.

From these examples of distorted beliefs, disputes, and sensible answers, we see that seemingly devastating predicaments aren't necessarily so when facts are separated from illogical assumptions and concerns.

Additionally, the CBT approach to alleviating everyday tiredness involves helping you see that it's in your best interest to experience short-term pain for the eventual benefits of long-term gain. You need to compare the advantages and disadvantages of tolerating momentary discomfort (for example, losing twenty pounds) for the sake of future gains (for example, feeling great). Increasing tolerance for frustration involves learning to challenge such debilitating thoughts as, "I'd exercise, but I mustn't experience physical discomfort! It's terrible if I do! I can't stand it!" while at the same time developing a more accepting attitude toward healthy lifestyle habits in general.

Thought Stopping

An effective technique to help you stop stressing over "the small stuff" is to use *thought stopping*. This means using a physical or verbal trigger to halt an undesirable thought. The trigger can be an action such as clapping the hands or snapping the fingers, or saying the word "stop" out loud. The trigger forces a clean break from the unproductive, disabling thought and paves the way for more practical thinking.

Once you become more aware of your unrealistic self-talk you can begin editing and controlling your internal voice to feed you with confidence-enhancing, sensible statements instead of critical, anxious, and guilt-producing ones. You'll want to make a deliberate effort to eliminate disabling thoughts and build on your best thoughts and emotions.

In short, first identify and challenge any unrealistic beliefs or expectations. Then use thought stopping. Let's try one:

1. *Cognitive Distortion*: "I'm trying to watch what I eat, but I've just got to have one of those donuts over there on the..."

2. *Thought Stopping*: "Stop!"

Here's another:

1. *Cognitive Distortion*: "I just have to keep everything spotlessly clean, or I'll catch germs and . . ."

2. *Thought Stopping*: "Stop!"

Easy, isn't it? It's also really effective!

Thought stopping is helpful when you have toxic thoughts that keep you from finding happiness, good health, and peace of mind. It helps teach you to stop those irrational thoughts by saying "stop" whenever a cognitive distortion comes to mind, followed by some time of intentional relaxation. You should use thought stopping whenever you're experiencing an increase in unwanted thoughts because you're focusing on them. Rest assured that as you continue to use this method, you'll discover how to acquire control over your cognitive distortions. The frequency of these thoughts will lessen with time. (If you still can't stop thinking about something, try distracting yourself. Exercise. Read a book. Watch a movie. Focus your attention on something or someone else.)

Practice, Practice, and More Practice!

Of course, psychological techniques like the ones described in this chapter are only techniques. To find long-term peace of mind, you'll probably have to work hard at changing your unhealthy thinking patterns. This means you'll want to *practice, practice, practice*. Why? Because when you practice a new activity, you effectively train it into your nervous system. We're sure you've learned to type on a keyboard or play a musical instrument. When you first begin to master a new skill like these, or any new skill, it all seems awkward. Your hands don't want to do what your head tells them to do. Every motion requires considerable conscious thought and effort to execute, and you can quickly become discouraged. Nevertheless, after many hours of practice, the new skill becomes more automatic, so that you no longer need to concentrate so intensely.

The same is true of learning and mastering cognitive reframing techniques. Once you've practiced and trained your nervous system into accepting this approach, you won't have to think about the techniques in order to use them. They'll become an instinctive reflex, available whenever you need them.

In his book entitled *Don't Believe It For A Minute! Forty Toxic Ideas that are Driving You Crazy* (1993), Arnold Lazarus and colleagues described it this way:

> One good rule of thumb: every time you catch yourself thinking a toxic or negative thought, make yourself consider at least two (more is better) positive self-statements or healthy counter-beliefs. This will help you work toward increasing psychological balance. At first this mental exercise might seem unnatural, but after a little practice, you will feel an increasing sense of familiarity with positive thoughts, making it progressively easier to achieve a more balanced mind and a winning and loving lifestyle (6).

At the end of this chapter is a Cognitive Reframing Chart to help you practice identifying and challenging the irrationalities in your life. Photocopy the chart, and whenever you recognize a personal cognitive distortion, record it and the situation in which it occurred. Then write your disputes and sensible replies. Also, try rating your level of distress both before and after you apply cognitive restructuring to your irrational thinking. Here's what a sample entry might look like:

1. *Situation*: Feeling guilty about not buying your kids the latest computer.

2. *Rating of Distress Prior to Cognitive Reframing* (1 = *least distress* to 5 = *most distress*): 5

3. *Cognitive Distortion*: "My kids will hate me if I don't buy them the latest computer."

4. *Dispute*: "What's the likelihood my kids will hate me?"

5. *Sensible Reply*: "While it's possible my kids will hate me, it isn't very likely. And even if they do, I can stand the discomfort."

6. *Rating of Distress Following Cognitive Reframing* (1 = *least distress* to 5 = *most distress*): 2

See how this works?

Finally, most people find it helpful to keep track of their practice sessions on paper, such as on the Cognitive Reframing Chart. With practice, you'll find it becomes easier and easier to dispute nonsensical thinking in your head without having to write anything down. For instance, you might catch yourself thinking you need to take on yet another project. However, instead of agreeing to do something that you can only squeeze in between 2 A.M. and 4 A.M., you'll automatically remind yourself that there's no external pressure to cave into someone else's demands.

Don't forget: cognitive therapy takes time, motivation, and self-reflection. But the rewards of rationality, simplicity, balance, and energy will definitely be worth your time and effort.

In Conclusion

Cognitive behavioral therapy uses a combination of techniques to reveal your root irrational and self-destructive philosophies, as well as show you what you can do to modify these. The goal in CBT, including REBT, is to help you accept reality, surrender your demands, and maximize your freedom of choice to find answers to your problems.

Don't get us wrong, though. Cognitive reframing isn't always easy to carry out. Changing long-term, deeply embedded patterns is tough, but it can be done with motivation and perseverance on your part.

In the next chapter, we present several other psychological methods used to restore everyday energy, particularly when exhaustion is the result of excessive amounts of stress.

Cognitive Reframing Chart

1. Situation:

Rating of Distress Prior to Cognitive Reframing (1 = least distress to
   5 = most distress):
Cognitive Distortion:
Dispute:
Sensible Reply:
Rating of Distress Following Cognitive Reframing (1 = least distress to
   5 = most distress):

2. Situation:

Rating of Distress Prior to Cognitive Reframing (1 = least distress to
   5 = most distress):
Cognitive Distortion:
Dispute:
Sensible Reply:
Rating of Distress Following Cognitive Reframing (1 = least distress to
   5 = most distress):

3. Situation:

Rating of Distress Prior to Cognitive Reframing (1 = least distress to
   5 = most distress):
Cognitive Distortion:
Dispute:
Sensible Reply:
Rating of Distress Following Cognitive Reframing (1 = least distress to
   5 = most distress):

4. Situation:

Rating of Distress Prior to Cognitive Reframing (1 = least distress to
   5 = most distress):
Cognitive Distortion:
Dispute:
Sensible Reply:
Rating of Distress Following Cognitive Reframing (1 = least distress to
   5 = most distress):

5. Situation:

Rating of Distress Prior to Cognitive Reframing (*1* = least distress to
    5 = most distress):
Cognitive Distortion:
Dispute:
Sensible Reply:
Rating of Distress Following Cognitive Reframing (*1* = least distress to
    5 = most distress):

6. Situation:

Rating of Distress Prior to Cognitive Reframing (*1* = least distress to
    5 = most distress):
Cognitive Distortion:
Dispute:
Sensible Reply:
Rating of Distress Following Cognitive Reframing (*1* = least distress to
    5 = most distress):

7. Situation:

Rating of Distress Prior to Cognitive Reframing (*1* = least distress to
    5 = most distress):
Cognitive Distortion:
Dispute:
Sensible Reply:
Rating of Distress Following Cognitive Reframing (*1* = least distress to
    5 = most distress):

8. Situation:

Rating of Distress Prior to Cognitive Reframing (*1* = least distress to
    5 = most distress):
Cognitive Distortion:
Dispute:
Sensible Reply:
Rating of Distress Following Cognitive Reframing (*1* = least distress to
    5 = most distress):

Feature:
Reframing Your Anger

We've all said, heard, and believed nonsense like:

"This-or-that makes me so mad!"

"So-and-so gets under my skin!"

"It's his fault, not mine!"

For the vast majority of us, a cosmic cause-and-effect force seems to control just about everything. Event A causes Thought B that causes Emotion C. As we've shown throughout *Stop Feeling Tired!*, events, thoughts, and emotions undoubtedly influence one another. But do events and your thoughts actually *cause* your emotions? Positively not!

Our premise here is simple: unbridled emotions—in this case anger—needlessly complicate your life. And this translates into stress, imbalance, and chronic tiredness. We believe it's our *perceptions* of events that determine our feelings and reactions, not the events themselves. To gain energy, we need to learn to manage our emotional reactions to the inevitable annoyances of life.

We're each in charge of how we interpret the events and people around us. It might seem like someone else is running your life, but your life really is your responsibility. And nowhere is this concept more obvious than with anger. Hence, your husband doesn't *make* you mad. You *choose* to let yourself get mad in response to something he said or did. It's not your employee's fault that you're miserable. You *decide* to be miserable. The broken VCR doesn't get you furious. You *opt* to be furious.

How do anger reactions happen in the first place? They follow a fairly typical pattern, which consists of four steps:

1. An event occurs in your surroundings.

2. You interpret the event as an "anger trigger."

3. You experience the emotion of anger.

4. You decide to express or not express your anger.

It's clear that all four steps in this anger reaction are related, but it's illogical to conclude that one or more of these steps positively *causes* the others.

What does this have to do with keeping your cool? You can learn to avoid exploding (avoid reaching Steps #3 and #4 above) by intervening at Step #2, the *thinking* step. Realistically, there's little or nothing you can probably do to stop Step #1 from happening, because life offers us plenty of occasions to lose it (some of these legitimate, others not). But there's a lot you can do at Step #2 to keep from progressing to Steps #3 and #4. Put another way, *you can change how you think about anger triggers*. You can see them at face value—irritations and nuisances that aren't worth getting upset about. And because it's only *lamentable* and not *horrible* when negatives happen, you don't *need* to react to them with aggression, even though this might be your first impulse.

Now for an example. Let's imagine that a disagreeable relative starts making biting remarks about your family. What happens? First, there are the remarks your relative makes (Step #1). Next, you listen to the remarks and interpret them as vicious assaults that you don't like (Step #2). Consequently, your blood begins to boil as you become overwhelmed by anger (Step #3). Finally, you decide that your relative's remarks deserve severe retribution, so you shout at him or worse (Step #4). Now, think about it: who's in control of your reactions in this case? Your relative? It might seem that way (and he or she might want you to think that!), but your relative isn't in control. You are! Whether or not you let malicious words get under your skin is up to you. You don't have to yell or lash out in revenge. There's no one forcing you to come out fighting.

Chapter 7

De-Stress Yourself

For fast-acting relief try slowing down.
—Lily Tomlin

One of our major themes throughout *Stop Feeling Tired!* has to do with the unique role that excessive stress plays in bringing about human misery. We'll even go so far as to claim that *stress is a primary operating factor in most mind-body problems.*

In a nutshell, we believe most chronic tiredness essentially results from too much stress, which results from the pressure that comes from not living simply. Here's an equation to illustrate:

complication → stress → *Qi* imbalance → everyday tiredness

The answer to chronic tiredness, then, becomes obvious. You need to lighten up on the chaos and hyperactivity in your life, which will reduce your stress. This, in turn, will reduce your *Qi* imbalance, which will reduce your chronic tiredness. Or, in equation form:

simplicity → calm → *Qi* balance → everyday energy

In this chapter, we consider some helpful tips for intervening at the stress stage of the equation in order to restore lost energy—a process we like to call *de-stressing*.

Stress Anyone?

According to most medical and psychological literature, the usual goal of de-stressing therapy is to help stressed out people (and their families) modify the kinds of thinking and behavior that reinforce and perpetuate undesirable physical symptoms, anxieties, depression, exhaustion, and so on. In the case of chronic fatigue, this means approaching life in a non-hectic way. When you think differently about how you're damaging yourself by overdoing everything, as well as decide to simplify and slow down, you can do a lot to minimize the life stresses that are wearing you down.

But before proceeding, a brief explanation of the nature of stress is in order.

Stress and the General Adaptation Syndrome

Stress, or the internal sense that your resources to cope with demands will soon be depleted, has recently received a great deal of attention in the area of applied psychology. Why has stress been studied so extensively? *Because the higher your stress levels, the more likely you are to develop physical symptoms or an illness*. We can all relate to stress, but the problem does seem to be particularly common among those who experience persistent tiredness.

Stress occurs in all age groups, although it seems to be increasingly inevitable with increasing years, given mortgages, career burnout, children, and aging parents. As one example of this, stress is keenly felt in adults who work. The most common sources of stress in the workplace include lack of expected progress (including promotions and raises), lack of creative input into decision-making, lack of challenging work, inadequate pay, monotonous work, feelings of being underutilized, vague job descriptions and procedures, conflicts with the boss or supervisor, lack of quality vacation time, workaholism, sexual harassment, forced career changes, and sudden job loss. In addition to an assortment of unpleasant physical symptoms (for example, migraines, ulcers, allergies), long-term job stress can eventually result in *burnout*, a state of mental exhaustion characterized by feelings of helplessness and loss of control, as well as the inability to cope with or complete assigned work.

Resistance to stress, known as *hardiness*, varies from person to person. Hardiness probably results from your adeptness at *cognitive appraisal*, or interpretation of stressors and the degree to which you feel able to control them, as well as your personality type, genetics, and lifestyle habits. For the most part, the reason we become stressed has a great deal to do with how we think about what's going on around us. Yes, past experiences can heavily influence us, but the mechanism of that influence is our thinking. For instance, if you were neglected as a young child, you might have the erroneous belief that you don't deserve to be happy or loved. In this case, it's today's belief that's bothering you, not the neglect from years ago. The point is that we have a substantial degree of control over ourselves and how we react to our circumstances.

In short, stress is unavoidable. But what you can change is how you look at and react to stresses in your life. Put simply, stress is really a "head" thing.

Experts often describe stress in terms of the *general adaptation syndrome*, which is explained in detail in Hans Selye's book, *The Stress of Life* (1976). Briefly, his model refers to the biological reactions that occur in response to sustained and unrelenting stress. Specifically, Selye has identified three stages in a typical stress reaction, with each stage leading to increased susceptibility to illness and even death. Selye's three stages are:

Stage 1. *Alarm:* When we experience a physical or emotional stressor, the body triggers an immediate set of reactions to counteract the stressor. Because the immune system quickly becomes depressed, our usual levels of resistance are compromised, which increases our susceptibility to infection. We typically recover rapidly when the stressor isn't severe or long-term.

Stage 2. *Resistance:* If, on the other hand, the stress continues, our immune system must work harder to keep up with the continued demands placed on it. For a while, we can become resistant to stress. But our resolve can't last forever. This is the time to combat the stress by practicing stress management or seeking a change in scenery. The problem at this stage is failing to do anything about our stress because we believe we're not susceptible to its effects.

Stage 3. *Exhaustion:* Because the human body is unable to maintain the resistance needed to battle long-term stress, we inevitably lose our resistance. Even though one person might be more or less resistant to stress than another, nearly everyone's immunity will eventually break down from prolonged stress. When this happens, organ systems and immunity begin to fail, and we fall victim to disease. Stress disrupts the natural balance—the homeostasis—that's crucial for our good health.

Most experts agree that Selye's general adaptation syndrome clarifies how stress can prove such an ample source of health troubles. Stress is one of the most significant factors in lowering resistance and triggering the various mechanisms involved in the disease process. However, by learning stress management and relaxation procedures, you can improve your chances of keeping your overall physical and psychological well being.

Virtually anything can be a stress trigger. For chronically tired folks, we often find an overloaded schedule, a hyperactive approach to life, unhealthy lifestyle habits, workaholism, and unhealthy thinking are some of the worst offenders. But one particularly nasty stressor has to do with not standing up for ourselves and saying *no* to all the pressures that modern life puts on us.

Assertiveness and Stress

In this section, we examine a lifestyle pattern that causes a great deal of stress for millions of Americans: *persistent lack of assertiveness*. It's one thing to pick your battles; it's another to feel like a doormat all of the time. When you don't stand up for yourself and say *no* to the demands of others, you end up agreeing to do things you don't want to, which wears you down. And before you know it, you're running on empty. Let's be honest—you have plenty to do without living someone else's agenda.

The Problem of Manipulation

Now take a moment and consider these soul-searching questions:

- Do you see yourself as a nonassertive person?

- Do you feel compelled to do what other people expect?

- Do you feel like people come to you for favors because they know you'll do what they ask?

- Do you feel like people push you around?

- Do you feel like people take advantage of your good nature?

- Do you hate the thought of making a scene in public for fear of what "they" might think?

If you can relate to one or more of these questions, you might have fallen into a pattern of nonassertiveness. Nonassertiveness, which we also refer to as excessive niceness, has to do with refusing to stand up for yourself when presented with others' requests, demands, pressures, and criticisms. Nonassertive people tend to be quiet and apologetic, worrying incessantly about offending others. They also tend to forfeit their own goals and needs in an attempt to please and appease everyone else. In contrast, assertive people set personal limits, take up for themselves, refuse to be manipulated, and make sure their own needs are fairly met. They also respect the rights of others to have their own opinions and take care of themselves.

You might be asking yourself, "Why do I let people run my life?" The answer might have something to do with your basic personality. For example, if you try to earn people's favor, yet feel constantly exploited and imposed upon, you're probably an *amiable* person. If so, you're always warm and friendly, work hard to avoid disagreements, grant favors, and give into others' requests. As an amiable person, you're likely to be nice, shy, and nonassertive.

Sadly, most nonassertive people are unhappy, stressed out, and drained. Why? One reason is that they intuitively know they don't deal well with modern life, which can be ruthlessly tough. Of course, there's nothing wrong with having concern for others and being charitable. If everyone were that way, our world would be a much kinder, gentler place. But that's not the way it works. So, it's not being nice that's really the problem, it's being *too* nice—nonassertive—that gets us into trouble.

You're only half of the problem, though, because it takes two to tango. The second reason nonassertive people are stressed out is that they too easily succumb to manipulation. That is, your non-assertiveness is a special problem when it's coupled with someone else's manipulation. If you're nonassertive, you'll need to work at being assertive to avoid being manipulated. Of course, we're not suggesting that you turn aggressive, angry, mean, demeaning, or sarcastic. None of this has anything to do with assertiveness. Rather, you can politely stand up for yourself at all times, especially when others want to take advantage of your niceness. In fact, we recommend being politely assertive whenever possible.

While you can't do much to change your basic personality, you *can* make changes in how you think, feel, and act. As you've already learned, the first step is identifying the culprits of your misery. Following are a few of the typical distorted thoughts that nonassertive folks believe when it comes to taking care of themselves:

- People must approve of me and my actions, so I can't disagree with them.

- Good people always assist others, no matter how unreasonable the demand is.

- I must always be gracious and helpful.

- It's rude to talk back.

- I can't challenge the way things are.

- I'd better move over when I'm pushed aside.

- If I tell someone just what I think, I might get angry or embarrass myself.

- What would the neighbors (or my coworkers, parents, etc.) think?

Contrary to what manipulators might want you to think, you don't have to buy into this kind of nonsense. As a human being, you're entitled to certain rights, such as:

- You have the right to say *no* and mean *no*.

- You have the right to set your own boundaries.

- You have the right to think for yourself.

- You have the right to find your own answers.

- You have the right to not know everything.

- You have the right to make mistakes and learn from them.

- You have the right to voice your opinion.

- You have the right to satisfy your own needs without feeling guilty.

- You have the right to keep to yourself if you want.

- You have the right to be imperfect and not live up to others' demands.

If you're a nonassertive person and want to protect yourself from manipulation, you'll want to start by transforming how you think about life. Change starts between your ears. Only by altering your thinking patterns will you be able to avoid the stresses associated with not standing up for yourself.

It's Good to Say No

One of the hardest words for nonassertive folks to say is *no*. This little word is emotionally loaded and carries lots of unpleasant associations. That's why so many nice, shy types hate to say it. They're afraid of being rejected, disappointing others, triggering an uncomfortable exchange—the list can seem endless. Stated another way, *no* means setting limits and standing your ground, and not everyone is willing or ready to do this.

Fortunately, it's easy to learn to say *no*. You just have to practice and then see that your world doesn't collapse when you refuse to budge. You can learn to say *no* with gusto and enjoy the peace of mind this tiniest of words can bring!

Saying No: Gently or Harshly?

We've had lots of experience saying *no*, although George tends to have more problem with this than Christie. Over the years, we've come to realize that a simple *no* is much more powerful (and far less trouble) than long, drawn-out excuse making. Consider this exchange:

Piper: Can I borrow your car?

Casey: Oh, well . . . uhh, the car's not really working, and it needs an oil change, and the insurance has lapsed, and the front left headlight is out, and the engine overheats. . . .

versus

Piper: Can I borrow your car?

Casey: No, I never loan out my car.

Get our point here? We'll take a short, assertive exchange any day over a drawn-out, nonassertive one!

We like to distinguish between two types of *no's*: *nice no's* and *blunt no's*. The former are cordial and gentle, whereas the latter are direct and to the point. We always prefer trying nice *no's* first, and then resorting to more direct *no's* as needed. We also find that people generally respond more favorably to nice *no's*—but this is our particular style. You'll have to decide what works best given your personality.

The point is that *you're being honest*, even if it comes across as harsh to the other person.

To be truly assertive, we believe, is to be honest, direct, and effective in our communications with others. Two of the most frequent forms of miscommunication patterns are psychological games and mixed messages. *Psychological games* are the roles and scripts people assume to keep from being themselves. By playing psychological games, people avoid dealing with personal and interpersonal issues and problems by not being straight with themselves or others. One example of a game is "I'm More Important," in which an individual has to "one-up" other people. Another example is "Pity Me," in which an individual continually complains to get attention. Game playing complicates relationships and if left unchecked, can make everyone involved miserable.

People also give *mixed messages*, of which there are three types. In the first type, the sender says one thing verbally, but says something entirely different with his or her body. An example of this is the employer who says, "I'm listening to you" while looking off in another direction. The second type of mixed message involves conflicting verbal messages, an example being the coworker who says in one breath, "I respect your opinion," and in the next, "Keep quiet!" In the third type, the sender says two different things with his or her body. An example of this is the boss who after being asked what she's feeling, says nothing, but smiles while clenching her fists.

One of the best ways to deal with psychological games and mixed messages (yours or anyone else's) is to accept the fact that they exist and to work at catching yourself and others whenever these faulty patterns arise. Of course, you should be careful when you point out to others that they're playing games. If you're tactful and keep at it, though, you'll eventually reap the rewards of direct, honest, open, and real communication.

De-Stressing

As bad as stress can be, you can learn how to eliminate a great deal of it from your life. We don't mean ridding yourself of all of life's pressures. As we've explained, these are inevitable. Think of it this way: pressure is what happens to you, and stress is your reaction to that pressure. The key to stress management, then, is changing the way you look at pressure—in other words, cognitive reframing.

Thankfully, de-stressing, or *stress management*, is a learnable skill. In the next section of this chapter, you'll learn about this and various

ways to reduce stress, as well as change your reactions to it. For start-
ers, you'll learn to:

- *Relax:* This helps your body learn how to "shut off" the "fight
  or flight" response. Relaxation methods (like PMR, described
  below) are based on the concept that you can't be apprehen-
  sive and relaxed at the same time. In essence, whatever you
  do that opposes the stress response will usually turn it off.

- *Practice deep breathing:* Take slow, deep breaths rather than the
  fast, shallow ones that most of us are accustomed to during
  times of stress.

- *Imagine a very peaceful scene:* Think of a real one or made-up
  one. Try to involve all of your senses as you imagine this
  relaxing place.

- *Develop social support:* Keep in mind that people with adequate
  social support networks report less stress and overall
  enhanced psychological health in comparison to those who
  don't.

- *Avoid stressful situations whenever possible:* Practice the cognitive restructuring techniques that form the basis of *Stop Feeling Tired!*

Cognitive Steps to De-Stressing

In the last two chapters, we discussed how cognitive methods
like rational-emotive-behavior therapy (REBT) can be so important for
managing stress and everyday tiredness. Let's quickly review how
CBT works.

In brief, you decide when and under what conditions your
thinking has turned dysfunctional. Once you've identified the source
of your irrational thinking, it's time to dispute and change your attitude in a way that creates rational thinking. Then, after a time of effective practice (you might experience positive changes within hours),
the problem or discomfort often goes away. In other words, *by altering
your irrational perceptions and replacing them with rational ones, it becomes
possible to recondition your mind to operate in newer, healthier ways.* The
process is summarized here:

- Use the Cognitive Reframing Chart found at the end of chapter 6.

- Discover your irrational thinking.

- Dispute and challenge your irrational thinking.

- Replace your distorted thoughts with sensible thoughts.

- *Practice, practice, and practice!*

In our opinion, this straightforward, cognitive approach to stress and exhaustion is the most effective for the most people. *Cognitive therapy is your first, best hope for de-stressing and overcoming everyday tiredness.* And while such psychological treatments as *insight therapies* (long-term therapies such as psychoanalysis) might have value in certain cases of everyday tiredness, we don't generally recommend them for everyday energy. However, we do recommend a number of behavioral therapies to help you retrain your mind by changing your behavior.

Behavioral Steps to De-Stressing

As behavioral specialists, psychologists have developed many effective techniques for de-stressing. In this section, we'll review some of these standard psychological therapies for stress and tiredness, with a focus on current methods that have been demonstrated to be the most useful.

The *behavioral perspective* holds that most, if not all, mental activity is directly related to behavior and learning. That's why *behaviorists*—clinicians who use behavioral techniques to treat problems—are primarily concerned with the roles that behavior and learning play in everyday living. Since the 1950s, many psychological problems (for example, stress, smoking, overeating) have been shown to respond favorably to treatment with behavior therapy.

Several of the more popular behavioral therapies that can be used to treat stress and chronic tiredness include *systematic desensitization* (which includes *behavioral analysis, relaxation training, deep breathing,* and creating a *graduated hierarchy*), *modeling therapy, exposure and response therapy, thought stopping and distraction, imagery and visualization, hypnosis, biofeedback,* and *homework assignments*. Not surprisingly, you can't perform many of these behavioral therapies without scheduling at least a few sessions with a licensed clinician. However, we want to give a brief overview of these methods in the event you decide to seek professional help for your chronic tiredness.

Systematic Desensitization

Whenever a pattern of mental, emotional, or physical behavior is *maladaptive* (interferes with successful functioning in your personal or social environment), the behavioral treatment of choice is *systematic desensitization*, also known as *graduated exposure*. Although psychologists typically recommend systematic desensitization to treat irrational fears, phobias, and anxieties, this behavioral technique has also been shown to be helpful for treating a wide range of other problems, including stress, tension headaches, muscle tension, alcoholism, drug abuse, depression, sexual dysfunctions, asthma, hyperacidity, and hypertension.

Joseph Wolpe developed systematic desensitization in 1958 when he became disenchanted with traditional psychoanalytical treatments. Wolpe discovered that an emphasis on exploring childhood memories and using Freudian "free association" was ineffective for treating soldiers with what was then called "war neurosis." Wolpe believed that his patients needed to be "deconditioned" because of their *learned* anxiety in association with traumatic situations. He then began to research and test his theory and later developed this powerful behavioral treatment.

The procedure of systematic desensitization consists of three basic parts: 1. A complete *behavioral analysis* of the client's situation, 2. *relaxation training*, and 3. *hierarchy construction* and *presentation*.

Behavioral Analysis. Behavioral analysis involves a complete psychological evaluation based on self-reports of behavior. In other words, behavioral analysis involves a therapist asking you about your stress and symptoms of tiredness, specifically in terms of how you respond to certain stimuli (the plural of "stimulus"). If your stress or tiredness disrupts your ability to function successfully in the world, behavioral analysis might prove beneficial.

Relaxation Training. When confronted with stressful situations, we often prepare ourselves to run or fight. This is known in psychology as the *fight or flight response*, which helps our bodies to reach a state of emergency-level readiness. If you've ever accidentally stepped off of a curb only to be almost hit by a car, you've probably noticed that your heart and breathing rates instantly and automatically increase. This is the fight or flight response in action; it's there to protect you—in this case, making you jump out of the way of the car. So, when you're in real, immediate danger, it's appropriate to feel afraid. Getting your body revved up with adrenaline could very well keep you alive.

The problem comes when we don't need this level of readiness—when running or fighting isn't needed. In other words, most of the time when we feel stressed, there's no imminent danger, so it's a false alarm. Put simply, the fire alarm is ringing, but there isn't a fire!

When the fight or flight response activates in the absence of a threatening situation, we typically experience anxiety or panic. Our modern-day lives keep us so busy that we're often too wound up. If our bodies remain in such a high gear state for long periods of time we can develop, in addition to anxiety, such bodily symptoms as headaches, tension, back pain, or stomach trouble. All of this drains us of our life energy. *Without a doubt, at least some of your symptoms of everyday tiredness are due to chronic high levels of stress.*

Many methods are available for learning to cope better with stress. One especially good method is learning to relax, which can help lessen the degree of useless physical arousal that most of us experience in today's fast-paced, hectic world.

Applied relaxation is now considered an established and efficient psychological therapy for stress, tension, worry, and anxiety. Applied relaxation can be just as effective as other behavioral methods, and can bring about significant improvements in nearly all cases.

Once your therapist determines that systematic desensitization is appropriate for you, you're taught techniques of *progressive muscle relaxation* (PMR), which involves the sequential contracting and relaxing of muscles. The goal is to assist you in achieving a feeling of muscular and mental relaxation. You start by relaxing your forehead and facial muscles, tensing these groups for a few seconds and then relaxing them. Next, you move down your body from your neck and shoulders to your shoulder blades, upper back, arms, hands, lower back, legs, and feet. You can also practice *deep breathing* (described below) during PMR by inhaling when you tense your muscles and then exhaling when you relax them.

Although you learn PMR in your therapist's office, you should practice it between sessions until you feel competent. You might also learn to use "SUDS" (*subjective units of distress scale*), in which you assign a numerical score ranging from 0 to 100 to the degree of stress you feel. The more stress or tension you experience, the higher will be your SUDS score. As you learn to relax, you should see your SUDS diminish.

Setting aside time to relax and get yourself "centered" can be of inordinate value in managing stress and ridding yourself of everyday tiredness.

Deep Breathing. As a natural energy boost, deep breathing exercises are another very easy way to relax your body. Most of us tend to fill only the upper chest when we breathe and thus miss how the increased oxygen intake relieves tension and improves metal alertness. Just notice how an infant's abdomen rises and falls with each breath. Now that's true deep breathing!

By using one or both of the deep breathing exercises provided below, you can quickly relax as well as potentially improve your circulation, oxygenate your blood, and strengthen your lungs.

Here's a really fast relaxation exercise for deep breathing, one that we frequently recommend:

1. Sit or lie down in a quiet place where you won't be disturbed for several minutes.

2. Recall some good, positive feelings.

3. Close your mouth and relax all of your muscles.

4. Slowly and deeply inhale through your nose (not your mouth) to a count of six or eight. As you do this, consciously push out your abdomen.

5. Hold your breath to a count of four.

6. Slowly breath out through your mouth (not your nose) to a count of six or eight.

7. Continue to repeat this "inhale-hold-exhale" cycle until you achieve maximum relaxation.

Still another relaxation method is known as *rapid relaxation*, in which you use stress-triggering thoughts as a cue to bring on a brief relaxation state. When you find your stress levels rising, take a couple of deep breaths, say the word "relax," and exhale. You should perform rapid relaxation while mentally scanning your body for tension and trying to relax everything as much as possible.

The Graduated Hierarchy. The next step in systematic desensitization involves creating a graduated hierarchy of your stressors or fears, ordered from lowest-arousing to highest-arousing situations. Completion of a hierarchy typically requires three to five sessions, although the process can take as little as one session or as many as twenty-five or more.

The final step in Wolpe's procedure is for a therapist to present the stressful situations in the graduated hierarchy first *covertly* (in the imagination) and then *overtly* (in real life). Meanwhile, during these "exposure" sessions, you practice PMR in response to each item on your hierarchy. In this way, you move step-by-step up your hierarchy as you become more at ease with whatever it is that stresses you out.

Let's take a look at some of the specifics of this procedure. First, during the covert portion of systematic desensitization, you're asked to relax and to visualize the least stressful item on your hierarchy. If you can imagine the scene without anxiety or tension for a minimum of ten seconds, the therapist presents the next item on the list. On the other hand, if you have anxiety or tension, you're directed to stop imagining the scene and tell your therapist all about it. Once you again become relaxed, you return to that item for a shorter period of time. Then you gradually increase your imagery times for that scene until you can easily visualize it twice in a row for at least ten seconds each. You continue this process until you're able to handle comfortably every item on your hierarchy.

Second, during the real-life (or *in vivo*) portion of systematic desensitization, you learn to transfer or "generalize" your reduced stress levels to real-life situations that are equivalent to the items on your hierarchy. *In vivo* practice is extremely important, because you reinforce in real life what you've learned in sessions.

Modeling Therapy

Stress can often be treated favorably with *modeling therapy*. In this procedure, you observe someone else (called the "model" or "actor") approach a stressful object or participate in a stressful activity that rings true for you (for example, having to return a defective piece of merchandise for a refund). The goal in modeling therapy is for you to relearn how to react under similar circumstances.

Although a live model is probably more effective, you can also watch a videotape of someone engaging in the activity. And if you have access to such technology, a virtual-reality session can also be a beneficial modeling tool. This technology uses computer-generated images and special headgear to simulate a realistic social environment that allows you to interact with it.

Exposure and Response Therapy

Unlike systematic desensitization that emphasizes relaxation while gradually confronting your stress, *exposure and response therapy* intentionally causes stress, tension, and anxiety. By repeatedly exposing yourself to a feared situation or object (either overtly or covertly), you experience such intense and sustained tension that it eventually loses its power over you.

Combining exposure with cognitive therapy appears to be very useful for some stressed-out, exhausted people.

Thought Stopping and Distraction

As you become more aware of your tendencies to engage in negative self-talk, you'll want to begin editing and controlling your "inner voice" in order to fill your mind with positive, confidence-enhancing self-talk rather than distorted thoughts of anxiety, shame, and self-criticism. You'll have to make a conscious effort to remove your distorted thoughts while building upon the attitudes and feelings that have characterized the happiest, most confident times of your life.

Thought stopping is an excellent way to eliminate negative self-talk. You'll recall from chapter 6 that this technique involves using a verbal or physical trigger to halt undesirable thinking. The most popular trigger is the word *stop*, said out loud or to yourself. You might even try screaming "Stop!" inside your head. You can also clap your hands, snap your fingers, squeeze your eyes tightly shut, think of a large red stop sign, or pop your wrist with a rubber band. Whichever you choose, your trigger allows you to break free from unproductive, debilitating thinking. Remember, you should be consistent in your use of thought stopping; use it every time you have irrational thoughts. As you continue to use this technique, you'll gain control of your thinking and watch the frequency of negative self-talk decrease.

Thought distraction involves shifting your thinking. One method is to think about something that's calming, such as a birthday celebration, a vacation you're planning, or a time when you felt delighted. Another method is to think about complex matters so that your mind becomes completely occupied. Two good examples are counting by seven (seven, fourteen, twenty-one, etc.) and saying the alphabet backwards in your head.

Don't forget that the more you practice these techniques, the better they work. In the beginning, it can be tough to shift your thoughts for more than a few seconds at a time. But with practice, thought stopping and distraction will become second nature to you.

Imagery and Visualization

Imagery, otherwise known as *guided imagery* or *visualization*, is used to change attitudes, behavior, or bodily reactions. It's well known that personality and consciousness are made up of mental images, and that to correct psychological problems, you have to identify and change these distorted images. In this way, guided imagery as a clinical tool involves your paying special attention to the specific images needed to bring about the changes in behavior that you desire. Imagery can be taught either individually or in groups, and a therapist will often use it to bring about a distinctive result (for example, less stress, improved diet, more exercise).

Practices that have a component of imagery are practically universal. These include systematic desensitization, REBT, biofeedback, hypnosis, neurolinguistic programming (NLP), gestalt therapy, and many others. In fact, any therapy that relies on imagination, visualization, or fantasy to communicate, motivate, solve problems, or increase awareness can be labeled a form of imagery. As well, forms of meditation that include reciting a mantra or focusing attention on an imaginary object can also be labeled a kind of imagery. Likewise, relaxation techniques and autogenic training can involve instruction (for example, "Your hands are heavy") that has a component of imagery.

Imagery consists of two major processes: *evaluation* and *mental rehearsal*. Evaluation involves asking you to describe your condition. You're literally asked, "How do you feel?" Mental rehearsal is then used to relieve stress prior to a stressful event (for example, having Christmas at your in-law's house). In most cases, a relaxation procedure is also taught, as are other coping techniques, like distraction and deep breathing. Mental rehearsal can lessen the discomfort and side effects associated with too much stress and chronic exhaustion.

Hypnosis

Hypnosis is as an altered state of consciousness (a trance-like state) in which susceptibility to suggestions is heightened and the recall of hidden memories becomes easier. A "hypnotic trance" is simply a very relaxed mental state, which can be reached through guided imagery and meditation.

Hypnotherapy relies on the use of suggestions to bring about personal change. More specifically, hypnosis involves an ability to set aside critical judgment without relinquishing it completely, as well as an ability to make-believe and fantasize. If you want to be hypnotized, you visit a clinical hypnotherapist and undergo *hypnotic induction*, in which you're instructed to relax and "go inside" your mind.

It's good to remember a couple of things about hypnosis. First, hypnosis isn't mind control or brainwashing. Second, the effectiveness of hypnotic suggestion has less to do with the skills of the hypnotist and more to do with the suggestibility and personality of the person hypnotized. Third, hypnosis can't cause you to act against your will or contradict your values. A hypnotherapist is ethically required to make only those suggestions that you've both decided are in your best interest. You won't be asked to do things against your morals or values. The idea that a hypnotized person is an automaton, is unable to resist any suggestion that's given, or won't be able to leave a trance is completely based on Hollywood-style misconceptions rather than facts. While hypnotized persons are susceptible to suggestion, there are very definite limits.

Hypnosis has many clinical applications and is well-documented as a therapy for mind-body problems. Given all of its benefits, hypnosis—especially when applied in combination with cognitive reframing—can be an exceptionally powerful tool for managing stress and treating everyday tiredness.

Biofeedback

Biofeedback is based on the principle that we have an innate potential to control with our mind, at least to a small degree, the autonomic functions of our bodies. For instance, you can be trained in a matter of hours or days to change the temperature of your hands, at will, by 5 or more degrees. You can learn to alter your brain waves, reduce the frequency of asthma or allergy attacks, or manage pain. You can even be trained to prevent a migraine headache. Various controlled trials and a number of field studies have shown that biofeedback therapy can effectively induce relaxation and reduce some of the complications associated with irritable bowel syndrome, tension headaches, and stroke. In other words, you can be taught to control the allegedly involuntary processes (for example, blood pressure, heart rate) that increase when you're under stress.

Biofeedback relies on special equipment with specialized sensors that track skin temperature, muscle contractions, and brain waves. The biofeedback machine "feeds back" your efforts at control in the form of a signal (for example, a buzz). Once you're connected to the biofeedback machine, you're instructed to extinguish the signal (which is often annoying). Because you have no idea what to do, you must rely on trial-and-error to determine how to relax and, thus, stop the signal. In this way, you eventually learn to control your responses to stress without the equipment. Most biofeedback sessions are scheduled weekly and last from thirty to sixty minutes.

Several different types of biofeedback machines can provide information about the systems in your body that are affected by stress. These include *EEG, EMG, GSR,* and *temperature feedback* machines.

EEG. An *electroencephalogram* (EEG) monitors brain wave activity. Because alpha waves are characteristic of states of relaxation (versus beta waves, which are characteristic of states of wakefulness), you might find relief from stress, muscle tension, anxiety, insomnia, and perhaps epilepsy by learning to increase your alpha wave activity. EEG seems to be more effective when used in combination with other methods like relaxation techniques and cognitive reframing. That way, you can learn how to control your reactions to stress while also exploring how your thinking and behaviors contribute to it.

EMG. An *electromyogram* (EMG) measures muscle tension. Two electrodes (or sensors) are taped onto your skin over the muscle to be monitored (for example, your jaw muscle). When the electrodes measure muscle tension, the device produces a buzz, beep, or colored light. You can hear or see continuous monitoring of your muscle's activity as you learn what tension feels like as it begins to mount. Then you can eliminate the tension before it worsens or causes physical problems. EMG seems particularly good for treating tension headaches, neck pain, jaw pain, backache, and stress-related conditions like ulcers and asthma.

GSR. *Galvanic skin response* (GSR) training (also termed "electrodermal response," or EDR) measures the skin's electrical conductance, which is related to sweat gland activity. You probably know this form of biofeedback from its use in "lie detector" tests. As a minute electrical current is applied to your skin, the GSR equipment measures changes in the levels of water and salt released from your sweat glands. The more emotionally aroused you are, the more active your sweat glands are, and the greater your skin's electrical conductivity is. GSR is frequently used for stress, tension, anxiety, phobias, panic, excessive sweating, stuttering, and poor athletic performance.

Temperature Feedback. This technique utilizes a machine that monitors skin temperature. A sensor is attached to a finger of your dominant hand or to a toe. If you're stressed out or nervous, your skin temperature will drop as blood redirects from your hands and feet to your internal organs and muscles. Temperature feedback can be invaluable for treating stress, migraine headaches, and circulatory disorders like Raynaud's disease (characterized by excessively cold hands and feet).

You can purchase small, inexpensive biofeedback instruments for use at home. The most affordable ones are designed to monitor only one response, such as your skin's conductivity.

Homework Assignments

If you decide to go into therapy to de-stress, your progress will depend largely on what you do outside of sessions. To assist you in making the most of any therapy experience, your therapist will probably assign you numerous homework assignments. At the start of each session, he or she will review your progress as reflected in these assignments.

It's normal not to want to do homework (try asking most teenagers!), but if you keep refusing to do as the therapist suggests, you might want to decide if, somehow, you're engaging in *self-sabotaging behavior*—getting in the way of your own progress by not properly engaging in your therapy. You might also want to consider what secondary gains you're receiving from not doing your homework. Always feel free to discuss any aspect of your homework assignments with your therapist.

Typical psychological homework assignments might include:

Written Assignments. Written homework assignments might take the form of keeping a journal, answering workbook questions, filling out your Cognitive Reframing Chart, or all three. You'll probably find it's easiest to set aside about thirty minutes every day to write out your homework assignments, which you'll then bring to sessions for your therapist to review.

Reading Assignments. Also referred to as *bibliotherapy*, reading is central to most therapeutic homework. Assignments might include reading books, articles, workbook materials, or information on the Internet. Reading, in and of itself, isn't probably sufficient to rid yourself of stress and restore your long-lost youthful energy. But it can be a great addition to other methods.

Experiential Assignments. It's not enough for most of us to simply think about our distorted beliefs. To eliminate long-held irrationalities, it's necessary to dispute them vigorously. In addition to doing this in your head, you must also try to act and emote rationally in your everyday life. Here are a few common REBT methods for accomplishing this:

- *Risk taking:* This involves taking risks by directly confronting your fears to eliminate them.

- *Attacking shame:* This involves countering embarrassment and shame by being silly—that is, doing something that would typically embarrass you but not hurt anyone else. Try making a spontaneous speech in the park, or break out into song while on the subway. These types of experiences will prove that you don't need others' approval or respect. In other words, when you see no one cares that you're being silly, you come to understand there's no need to worry about what others might be thinking.

- *Attacking perfectionism:* Here you battle your perfectionistic tendencies by purposely doing things imperfectly. Some good examples are shaving only part of your face, not making your bed, leaving dirty dishes in the sink, and not washing your car after driving through mud.

- *Discomfort tolerance:* You subject yourself to unpleasant, annoying situations to practice not upsetting yourself. A good example is intentionally driving into a huge, tangled traffic jam to learn frustration tolerance.

Many people express strong feelings—from boredom to apprehension to excitement—when it comes to doing these sorts of homework assignments. It's best to discuss your feelings openly with your therapist. Although homework assignments can be uncomfortable or downright frustrating, you find you receive much more from therapy if you take the time to do them.

Therapy Formats

We also want you to know that the methods described in this chapter can be taught in various formats. The two most popular are individual therapy and group therapy, both of which differ from self-help therapy.

Individual therapy typically includes weekly one-on-one meetings with a psychologist, psychiatrist, counselor, social worker, or other mental-health professional. This type of therapy provides you with a chance to process such important issues as anxiety, stress, depression, self-doubt, dissatisfaction, shyness, sexual and relationship problems, family conflicts, educational difficulties, drug and alcohol abuse, eating disorders, or virtually any other concern. Most of us have been troubled by concerns like these at one point or another in our lives. If you're experiencing significant discomfort that requires help beyond the suggestions provided in this book, you should consider seeking personal counseling. There's no reason to feel embarrassed. Going in for some individual therapy is perhaps the most responsible step you can take to rid yourself of chronic tiredness, as well as most any other psychological problem.

Group therapy typically includes weekly meetings with one or two mental health professionals and a small group of clients. The idea is to work toward understanding and resolving various concerns within a group context. Whereas you might believe your problems can best be addressed in individual counseling, a therapy group's support, input, and feedback can be unparalleled in terms of helping all members develop awareness and overcome life hurdles. How? In group therapy, you have an opportunity to examine your reactions to a range of people, to experiment with new ways of interacting, and to give and receive feedback.

One special form of group therapy is *couple's therapy* or *relationship counseling*, which is designed to deal with conflicts or relationship problems peculiar to spouses or partners. Generally speaking, a couple meets together with their therapist for weekly sessions. Many couples have had their relationship damaged by one person's chronic tiredness and thus find it helpful to seek relationship counseling.

In Conclusion

In this chapter, we've introduced you to a wide range of methods for conquering your stress. Each technique can be used alone or in combination, though many require the expertise of a licensed clinician. *We've repeatedly found that starting with self-help cognitive therapy methods is best, following with behavioral methods when the situation warrants it.* Try solving your problems on your own first, and then seek professional help if you feel you need more.

If you ever experience problems being assertive, this chapter should also be good news. By mastering and applying our techniques, you can take charge with confidence in your ability to handle and stand up for yourself in virtually every situation. You'll quickly regain control of your life, and you'll feel less stress and more energy.

FEATURE:

DON'T GET PSYCHED OUT BY TECHNOLOGY!

"No matter what I do, my e-mails keep bouncing back."

"I get that stupid message, 'Your computer has performed an illegal operation.' What the heck does that mean—the FBI is going to confiscate my PC?"

"I spend more time fixing my computer and the company's network than using them. I'm about ready to go back to writing on yellow pads!"

"You need an electrical engineering degree to operate our office's thermostat!"

We've all experienced it—computerized technology that doesn't function properly. PCs that crash on Monday morning, copiers that melt transparencies, printers that smear ink on Board reports, phones that crackle during crisis calls, Internet viruses that destroy everything but non-essential data, fax machines that send documents to the wrong long-distance number, and so forth. The litany is nearly endless.

As we've described throughout this book, many strategies exist to help you deal with difficult or even "impossible" life situations, including those in which technology seems to have gone awry. Here, we present you with some insights into living a peaceful coexistence with computerized gadgetry.

Let's examine some of the crazy-makers and disputes for a typical person who lets himself get really annoyed, for example, when he can't make his e-mail program work. Try these beliefs on for size:

- My email mustn't do anything to frustrate me, because that'll be disastrous, and I'll hate work and life in general.

- I must be free to do whatever I want easily whenever and wherever I wish; otherwise, life is unbearable and I can't be happy at all.

- It's horrible if people think I'm dumb or disapprove when I can't figure my e-mail program out. If they dislike me, then their disapproval is intolerable. And it's always catastrophic if people think less of me.

- My self-esteem is completely tied up in my technology. If it doesn't work flawlessly, then I'm automatically inadequate and worthless.

And now for some sample disputes and sensible answers:

- Where's the law that says I mustn't ever be frustrated?

- It's inconvenient if I can't get what I want, or if people treat me badly, but it certainly isn't terrible. I can stand it, just as I've done many times in the past. No matter how poorly my e-mail functions or other people act, I can still keep my cool and accept myself the way I am.

- Sometimes life stinks! But that's no reason for me to get upset about it. Tomorrow always brings a new day.

- Who says people have to like me, accept me, or praise me? What counts is the fact I feel comfortable with myself and my abilities.

- I'm a fallible human being who makes mistakes. My self-worth isn't dependent on others' opinions of me or on my mastery of anything. And it doesn't matter if people think there's something wrong with me. It might be nice, but I don't *need* their approval!

Get the idea? Let's try a few more reframes. To get rid of those nonsensical ideas involving your having to like and get along with your fax machine, or the terribleness of losing your self-respect if you can't program your television's remote control:

1. First, identify your *crazy-makers*:
   - I *must* enjoy working with gadgets.
   - I *must* keep up with, purchase, and master the latest version of everything—computer processors, software, wireless contraptions, universal remotes, CD burners, etc.
   - I *must* always be 100 percent in control of the technology in my life.

2. Next, consider how demanding *musts* inevitably lead to *catastrophizing*:
   - If I don't like gadgets, it'd be horrible.
   - If I don't keep up with, purchase, and master the latest version of everything, I'll look stupid in front of my boss (coworkers, employees).
   - If I don't always control the technology in my life, then I'm a failure and an awful person.

   . . . and how demanding leads to the experience of low frustration tolerance:
   - If life is horrible and I'm a failure and a screw up as a person, then I won't be able to stand it.

3. Third, make up several *disputes* that challenge your nonsensical thinking:
   - So what if I don't like gadgets? What's so horrible about that?
   - Why do I always need to master everything? If for some reason I don't, why does that mean I'll look stupid?
   - Where's the rule that says if I don't control the technology in my life then I'm a failure and a screw-up?

4. And finally come up with some *sensible answers* to your disputes:
   - It's inconvenient if I don't like or get along with my gadgets, but it isn't horrible.

- It may be uncomfortable when I don't always own and master everything I want, but that doesn't mean I'll look stupid.

- It's unfortunate if I can't control my technology, but there isn't any rule that says I'm a failure because of this.

To find true and lasting happiness with computerized technology, you'll want to work at changing your irrational thinking patterns into rational ones. In the end, it's important to keep in mind that what probably bothers people the most about technology is the frustration that typically accompanies its breaking down. And the best means of dealing with this frustration? *Don't get psyched out!* Instead, try accepting computers and other electronic wizardry for what they are—fallible mechanisms.

CHAPTER 8

LIVE SIMPLY

*Everything should be made as simple as possible,
but not simpler.*

—Albert Einstein

As this quote from the twentieth century's most famous genius and scientist reminds us, simplicity in life is desirable. No doubt, the more you simplify your life, the less stress you'll feel and the more energy you'll have. But, as we discuss in this chapter, a lot of well-meaning folks take "simple living" to an impractical extreme. That's no good either.

As we've said throughout *Stop Feeling Tired!*, we believe in a balanced approach to life—one that avoids extremes. Let's face it, extremes of any type can drain you. One scoop of ice cream tastes delicious, but fifteen scoops will make you sick. And if you're really and truly craving ice cream, avoiding it completely will leave you feeling deprived.

The same thing applies to simplicity. It's okay to watch some television, read an occasional magazine, and treat yourself to a donut. But we're sure you'll agree that your life is out of balance when you have the television blaring at top volume all day, read nothing but Hollywood gossip columns, and gorge on an entire dozen donuts at one sitting. It's also stressful to utterly refuse yourself an occasional pleasure if something is really important to you.

So, yes, your life "should be made as simple as possible, but not simpler." Go slowly, and make reasonable changes that won't make you feel like you've moved into a refugee camp.

The Maintenance of Daily Life

Have you ever thought about how long it takes just to live life and take care of stuff? Well, let's think about it for a minute. First, just taking care of our bodies takes a considerable amount of time and energy. There's the daily routine of showering, grooming, and dressing, coupled with all the other things we do to keep our bodies in a socially acceptable form.

If we're behaving as we should be, there are dental appointments every six months, annual physicals and eye exams, as well as aerobic workouts and weight-bearing exercises at least three times per week. Then there's the endless need for errands: packages to the post office, prescriptions from the pharmacy, kids to doctor, pets to the vet, clothes to and from dry cleaning. Of course, we can't forget hair cuts, obligatory shopping (that is, for groceries and toothpaste), and oil changes (and don't forget to check your tire pressure once per month). Living generates costs, costs are bills, bills take time to pay, and checking accounts take time to balance. All this living makes a mess, which requires house cleaning, washing dishes, and doing laundry. Don't forget to check those smoke alarms and service those fire extinguishers regularly! Those of us who are home owners have yards, lawns, gutters, and houses that need maintenance. Furnaces need filter changes every month, chimneys need annual servicing, and all the tools we use to take care of the house and yard need regular maintenance—don't forget to properly service your lawn mower every spring! Then we have taxes, birthdays, church and social events, other holidays, and an endless array of activities with the kids. But above all, don't forget to eat right and get eight hours of sleep every night. Yeah, right.

Those are just the basics, not counting hobbies, vacations, and other entertainment—the stuff we *want* to do. It's no wonder that things go undone, things break because they weren't properly taken care of, and we don't feel our best because we haven't taken care of ourselves. What should we do? Simplify and organize. Disorder adds to complexity; organization leads to simplicity.

Needs Versus Wants

We can't escape the fact we live in one of the most affluent societies to have ever existed in the history of the world. What we accept as commonplace would be seen as wild extravagance in other places throughout the world. We don't just have running water, we have multiple bathrooms with massaging shower heads. We don't just have transportation, we have cars with our every comfort possible: air conditioning, bucket seats, cup holders, entertainment. We don't just have clothing, we have wardrobes so extensive that most of us have a hard time finding homes and apartments with closets big enough, and new construction accommodates ever-larger walk-in closets. We don't just have food to meet our nutritional needs, we have every conceivable culinary and junk-food luxury. It's gotten to the point that the greatest health problem in America today is obesity, leading to what health experts are now calling an epidemic of diabetes and other obesity-related conditions.

Our expectations of what we need has been transformed by living in a world of corporations ready to sell everything we want, and even those things we don't yet know we want. We have a culture that doesn't want, in *any* way, to be deprived. We have generations of people acclimated to the attitude that they should never suffer any discomfort or inconvenience. Food should be instantly available everywhere to suit our every whim, and any ache or pain or fever should be instantly relieved with a pill or potion. As a culture, we abhor that which discomforts us.

As we satisfy our ever-increasing desire for things, we unnecessarily complicate our lives. As we've seen, having and tending to things takes time and space. The hardest part is learning to determine what we really *need* versus what we *want* very, very badly. And it seems we always want just a little bit more than what we can honestly afford (more on that in the next section). If properly maintained, most modern vehicles will last for nearly 200,000 miles before needing major engine work. Why do we dump them every three or four years for the latest, biggest thing? The truth is, however much we protest that we don't compete with the Jones', we're keenly aware of what others have. We're also easily enticed by the newest, latest, brightest models that auto makers roll under our noses.

Beyond this, we feel compelled to acquire every doo-dad and gadget that comes along. Knickknacks, trinkets, endless accessories, kitchen and other household gizmos—the possibilities are as endless as the ads that bombard us everyday. And somehow, way too much of this stuff finds its way into our lives and into our homes. We see it, convince ourselves we need it, rationalize it, justify it, then it adds to the disorganization and clutter of our lives. The way to get control is to get organized.

Getting Organized

For many, getting organized is an overwhelming thought. You may see the mountains of clutter and disorder, stuff strewn about your home, stuffed in closets, jammed in drawers that resist opening, and not know where to start. You may have thoughts of simply moving away, leaving everything behind and starting over! Or, as George has fantasized: put it all in a U-Haul truck and drive it over a cliff. We know some who have threatened to do just that, as it would be easier to start over than plow though the disarray of life. Take heart—even the most organized among us have felt this way at one time or another.

The key to being successful in completing any large or overwhelming task is breaking it down into its parts. What makes something overwhelming is looking at the whole of it. Anything taken as a whole can seem huge—too huge to deal with. The other thing that makes a large task overwhelming is that at first it resists being broken down into parts. It's often hard even to know where to start. There's no obvious Step One, no place that presents itself as a logical beginning. And often when we decide where to start, it suddenly seems something else needs to be done first. We get caught in a quagmire of doing this before we can do that, and the next thing we know we're derailed entirely, throwing our hands up in futility.

If you try to jump in one weekend and organize everything, you may set yourself up to fail. The chaos of our lives generally defies such sweeping reform, making this the fastest route to being overwhelmed and failing—not to mention driving your family crazy. As with most things, the way to get organized is to make a plan; in other words, be organized about getting organized.

Make a list of all the things you think are disorganized, aren't being done as they should, or in any way frustrate you. Don't think about how you'll ever get these things done, and don't allow yourself to consider any self-defeating talk. Focus only on how you'd like your life and living space to exist in a an ideal reality. You may want to walk around your home, look in cupboards, closets, desks, storage areas. What do you have a hard time finding? What have you had to search for lately? What's hard to get to? Unused? In the way? What are those things that you think you should get to "one of these days," but you just haven't gotten to yet?

Maybe the things you want to organize are less tangible, like your schedule or your finances. Whatever it is in your life that you'd like to organize, put it on the list. If you're honest with yourself, the list will grow discouragingly long.

Next, prioritize your list. Your first impulse may be to put the biggest job as the highest priority, but that may not be the best approach. If you're easily discouraged or derailed from getting organized, maybe it would be better for you to prioritize your list by what would be easiest to do, or what would make you feel the best; that is, what task would make you feel better about yourself and your accomplishments? What would give you the best return on your time investment? It may be that one of the smaller items on your list may have a greater impact on day-to-day life, and would give you more satisfaction than accomplishing a bigger job. In other words, cleaning out and organizing your desk at home may be more satisfying than cleaning the whole garage. This would be a better place to start, as it'll get your momentum going.

Another method recommended by Janet Luhrs in *The Simple Living Guide* (1997) is to use the "drawer-by-drawer, shelf-by-shelf rule." She agrees that the organizing task can be overwhelming, but has added:

> If you look at your entire house as one unit of junk, you'll never do anything because the job is too overwhelming. Take it one drawer at a time. Start anywhere. Pick one room and work around in a circle until you've gone through the entire house. Take each room shelf by shelf, drawer by drawer (355).

Even so, we recommend you list and prioritize the rooms to keep yourself on task and to be sure to get the whole job done. Once you've made the list, assign each task a day or time to be worked on. You've probably heard the saying, "A place for everything, and everything in its place." While that's true of organizing things, it can also be said, "A time for everything and everything in its time." Whatever you want to get done will only get done if you plan to do it and make time to follow that plan.

If you've been honest with yourself and listed everything that needs attention, scheduling to get it all done may go farther into your future than you can reasonably plan. The solution to this is simple: plan only about a month or two worth of organizing projects at a time. Group the remaining items on your list together, and at the end of your planning schedule, set aside time to plan the completion of the remaining tasks. Set aside time to finish planning when you have a better idea of your schedule. That way, the things you need to do are still on the radar, but are in a holding pattern.

In keeping with our themes of energy, simplifying, and balance, we also recommend that, in planning your organizing schedule, you plan time for relaxation and rewards along the way to keep you motivated. All work and no play is another sure formula for failure.

Clutter

The myth: cleaning up clutter and staying organized takes a lot of time and is hard to do. Reality: absolutely *not true*. The truth is the exact reverse—getting rid of clutter and staying organized takes far less time and energy than living in a mess.

Okay, we'll confess: we're self-proclaimed "neat freaks." We both hate clutter, though Christie can tolerate a week's worth of mail piled up on her desk until she gets to it on the weekend, when it's promptly sorted and dealt with. On the other hand, George's ideal is a minimalist's fantasy inspired by a previous New York editor of his: a desk populated with only a blotter and a pen.

While some people out there are neat freaks for the sake of being neat, we like to keep things neat, papers under control, and stuff put away in its own place because we're busy, and keeping it all organized does, without doubt, save us time and energy.

Clutter, in and of itself, creates stress. Papers and stuff on desks, counters, or spilling across the floor speak of things not done, or too much unused, unneeded stuff. Such disorder also results in the loss of important papers or other items, time spent searching for those items, lost or late payments of bills, and general stress because a simple life task has been made harder only because there wasn't an orderly process set up for it.

That being said, we recognize that some people organize by files, others by piles. We advocate files—though we have friends whose piles are absolutely organized to them, and they can find anything in roughly a minute or two. For those of you who fit that category, we challenge you to convert your piles into files. If it can be stacked vertically on a desk or counter top, then it can be filed in a filing cabinet just as easily and accessibly. Or, as one friend of ours does, you could put your neat piles into contained cubby holes in your office space, one cubby hole per project. Using this system, our friend knows exactly where everything is.

Then there are those whose clutter is just disorganization, plain and simple. And that would describe most of the clutter in the world.

Clutter starts with one thing put on the counter or table. One newspaper, one stack of mail, one thing that doesn't have it's own place to live. Once one thing hits the counter, it's easier to put the second, third, etc. with it. In short, clutter multiplies. Clutter begets clutter. But, if the counter or table stays clear, then that one item stands out, and we can better resist putting that something on the counter where it doesn't belong.

Much of our clutter is caused by what is now being termed "affluenza." Once again our prosperity catches up with us. We have more stuff because we can, not because we necessarily need much of it. Can you imagine someone from Somalia or Afghanistan having a problem with clutter? Not likely. Clutter is a by-product of modern living and consumerism run amok.

Gurus on methods to simplify living have written entire chapters, yes, even entire books on getting rid of clutter. What they all point to is how much stuff we have that we never use and all the irrational reasons we have for hanging on to those things. We convince ourselves that we'll someday use that gadget, or we resist throwing it out or giving it away because we remember all too well how much we paid for it. We don't really want to admit to ourselves that we were duped into buying something that we haven't used, or used once or twice and will never use again. So we stash that thing into a closet, cupboard, garage, or attic. When we've collected way too many of such things, we rent a storage unit. Tsk. Tsk. As a friend of George's remarked:

> What's a family supposed to do these days? People, especially relatives and friends, give us stuff we don't want or need. We've really gotten to dread the holidays. Junk, junk, and more junk. The stuff piles up, but you can't get rid of it because the gift-givers will get their feelings hurt. Believe it or not, we've had friends actually ask to see a gift they gave us years before. And then there's all the junk we buy. Also, we hate to get rid of all the useless heirlooms. We finally rented a storage unit to store our boxes. There are days when the weather man on TV is talking about tornadoes or hurricanes. Deep down, the thought of everything getting blown away to the Land of Oz sounds pretty appealing!

While we believe that we should be more critical about what we keep, we also object to the extreme methods proposed by some authors for getting rid of clutter (including subjecting your belongings to the fury of Mother Nature!). Some experts would have you cancel all magazine subscriptions, get rid of the TV, and eliminate every gadget from your home. After reading some of their books, we honestly wonder what these people do once their clutter is gone!

We advocate being reasonable and honest with ourselves. Keep the magazines you do take the time to read (be *honest*: do you *really* read them?), reduce the number of hours spent watching TV (be honest: how many times do you look for something to watch instead of turning the TV off?), and get rid of the gadgets you don't use. Maybe, just maybe, the reason you don't use some gadgets is they're hiding behind a mess of other stuff. If they were accessible, they might be used more often.

One of the most common recommendations is to get rid of anything you haven't used in a year. This is generally a good rule for wardrobes, gadgets, and things lurking in garages and attics. But we see this as a reasonable rule of thumb, not an absolute dictate. We happen to be people with a number of hobbies: gardening, sewing, playing music, and reading books, among others. We have walls upon walls of books and magazines, some of which we haven't looked at in years. Many organizers would have us throw these out or give them away. They point out that these resources are available at the local library. This may be true, and in many cases we've gotten rid of magazines that we can access online or at the library.

But get rid of them all? We disagree. Many of those books and magazines have gone out of print and aren't available at libraries, which tend to clean out their clutter to make way for newer materials. We also don't want to run to the library every time we want to refer back to a magazine article, as we often do for the writing projects we work on. Getting rid of everything would mean an errand to the library, another errand that takes us away from home. That complicates life. It's easier to go to our own private library. But therein lies the secret. Although we keep these books and magazines, they're organized, and we can find what we want quickly. No rummaging. No going through boxes in a storage unit. We've gotten rid of the ones we won't use and have neatly kept the ones we do. We've sought the best of both worlds: we have the things we want and keep them accessible, but we get rid of excess clutter.

Those with less discipline for organizing themselves and staying organized do need to be more rigorous about getting rid of things, we admit. But if you've led a life in the extreme of clutter and keeping too much stuff, we caution against going to the other extreme. Balanced, reasonable living is our mantra. Extremes in either direction, we argue, end up making us crazy.

Besides the dump-it-in-a-year-if-you-don't-use-it rule, the other most-often quoted rule is that of equilibrium. This one we find more agreeable. This rule advocates that when you get a new item, a similar, older one must go so that you maintain the same volume of stuff, or an equilibrium. For example, if you buy a new pair of shoes, get rid of an old pair. Make a certain space in your closet for shoes, and only have as many as fit in that space neatly and accessibly. In contracting the disease of affluenza, we've convinced ourselves that we never have enough shoes, clothes, accessories, etc. We want our collection of stuff to make us feel better, assuming that the more of it we have, the better we'll feel about ourselves. Unfortunately, the reverse is true: the more stuff we collect, the more we've paid, and the harder we've worked to make the money to pay for it. When much of this stuff ends up being stressful clutter, we wind up feeling worse about ourselves and have only the vaguest idea why.

Except on rare occasions, when we bring something home, something else goes out. We'll stay within our space and will not, *will not* succumb to the lure (and unnecessary expense) of a storage unit.

If you want the best all-around resource we've found for getting yourself and your home organized, then we strongly recommend www.organizedhome.com, apparently the brain-child of Cynthia Townley Ewer. For every possible thing you could conceive of organizing, she has found a method to organize it, and she makes those strategies available for free. And we find her approach reasonable. This comprehensive Web site offers a multitude of resources both on- and offline. We'll share some highlights with you here to better motivate you to check out the site itself.

First, in a Web page titled, "A Tightwad's Guide to Getting Organized," Ewer explained:

> Organization is a process, not a product. It involves time and thought, motivation and effort—and you can't buy these factors in any store. No tangible item, no matter how useful, can set you on the road to better organization all by itself. The moral is: nobody ever got organized by buying stuff. Instead, they ended up holding a yard sale (online article).

We couldn't have said it better ourselves. Organization is a method of simplification, not a matter of complication by buying more stuff. If your first impulse is to run out to your local home-improvement store and buy closet and wall unit organizers, restrain yourself. Before you can organize anything, you have to figure out what you're going to organize. Chances are, once you've honestly gone through most of the stuff, you can simply get rid of it. Have that yard sale. With what's left, as Ewer suggests, measure first. Figure out how much space the item to be stored takes, and measure the space where you plan to put it. Then go buy what you really need to set up orderly storage—that is, if you still need to purchase anything at all.

Staying Organized

If you follow all of our wonderful advice and get yourself beautifully organized but don't change your long-term habits, then the organizing will have been for naught. If you want the benefits that come with simpler living and less clutter, then you have to change the habits that created the clutter in the first place. That way you stay organized.

The best way to keep organized is to set reasonable expectations; that is, realize that organization is not a one-time event, but a way of living. Organization doesn't magically happen. Just as it takes planning to get organized, likewise it takes planning to *stay* organized. While this sounds more complicated, the reverse is true. Once you get into the habit of organization, it creates its own momentum. In the end, it makes your life simpler, leaving you the energy to do more things that you want to do while giving you a better sense of calm and serenity.

The common temptation, the bad advice we give ourselves, is that it takes too long to stay organized. Once again, the opposite is true. The minute or two up front that it takes to put something away where it belongs, saves much more time down the line. It takes less time to clean up a mess before it's made than after. Our greatest challenge to staying organized is challenging our own perceptions and our tendency to lethargy and disorder. It's usually outright laziness that says "I'll get to it later," and this generally means not getting to it at all. The temptation to put it off most likely comes when we're tired. Maybe you've had a bad week at work, a week of extra demands. Maybe you're getting a cold. That's when good intentions slip.

Yes, we admit, even being the neat freaks we are, this happens to us, too. The difference is, we may let things slip a day or two, sometimes as long as a week if things get really awful. But after that we stop and take the time and get things back on track.

The other key to staying organized is paying closer attention to our habits and to exactly those moments when our organization starts to fray. We often lead distracted lives, doing one thing while our minds are on another. We don't, then, pay attention to when we take that first step toward undoing all our organization. Organization-loving person that she is, Christie's toughest challenge was keeping drawers of socks and nylons tidy. Try as she might, no matter how many time she organized them, they fell into disarray. While no one ever sees inside these drawers, and many might argue, "What difference does it make?" Christie would argue that it made a huge difference. She was losing as much as five minutes every morning and experiencing the untold stress and frustration of trying to find what she wanted while getting ready for work. So what? you say. That five minutes every morning amounts to twenty-five minutes a week, or about 1,300 minutes per year, or 21.66 hours per year. Almost one full day of her life every year all because a couple of sock drawers weren't organized. Life is too short as it is without letting disorder make it shorter.

What Christie did was organize her sock drawers one last time. First she threw out about half that she never wore. She folded and organized the rest, putting smaller items in a decorative box neatly containing them. Then she watched. She watched her own habits to see at exactly what point they became disorganized. It wasn't in the morning when getting ready. It was when she was putting away laundry. Things were getting shoved in quickly, causing disorganization and the resulting morning rummage.

By getting rid of the unneeded and by taking a matter of seconds, not minutes, longer while putting away laundry, Christie has added nearly a day to her life every year—a day to spend reading or doing what she wants rather than plowing stressfully through a mess of things she doesn't need. That's what we mean by simplifying and organizing to gain time and energy. When we adopt such simple habits, we find we're ultimately more rested, feel less stress, and are in better, reasonable control of our lives. Finally, we control our things rather than letting our things control us.

Planning Ahead

The world we live in, given its seemingly ever-increasing pace, demands that we attend to things in the moment, though, ironically, we're often robbed of living in that very same moment. The other irony is, by stepping back and planning better for the future, we can simplify and better seize the moment. Our approach is realistic: by default the world we live in requires a certain level of complexity. However, much of the complexity we bring on ourselves, and insofar as possible, we can reduce or eliminate that. For the rest, for the unavoidable residue of what we must deal with in order to live in the world today, the way to simplify it is to organize it. The way to organize it is to plan it.

Trying to remember everything is futile. But just writing it all down won't necessarily help either. The written form needs to be predictable, coherent, and legible. We're thinking here of a family with a number of people going in multiple directions, all needing to be clothed in clean clothes, fed, and provided with reliable transportation to and from the places they need to go. The only way to pull that off is if everyone knows what is expected and when.

Old-fashioned methods call for wall calendars and message boards. If this is your chosen method, look in office supply stores for the erasable wall calendars where you write in the dates. These are cheaper in the long-run, and you can get them big enough to handle all the family activities.

Many savvy families today are going high tech. While this doesn't sound at first like simplifying your life, done carefully, within reason and control, technology *is* capable of simplifying our lives. Resources are available to set up family networks with calendars and electronic message boards. We see no reason for a corporate-quality network server and computer system here. A basic computer with standard organizing software set up in a central home location will do. The key here is getting everyone to check in regularly, post their activities, and read the messages. Given most kids' fascination with computers, it won't be difficult getting them on board with the plan.

The point is simply doing it. Get in the habit.

Money and Debt

Of course, our perspectives on what we need and want translate into our finances. Financial concerns are a major source of stress, and indeed, remain the leading cause of divorce. Suzie Orman, a leading personal financial guru, points out that we're taught reading, writing, and mathematics, but not the basics of personal finance and budgeting. In short, most of us don't handle money well because we've never been taught how to do so. We live paycheck to paycheck without the benefit of long-term planning. Or, we think if we contribute to a 401K plan through our employer that we've done what is necessary to plan for the future.

Not only do we buy things to start with, we pay to maintain or store them. They don't just cost us on the day we buy them, but they cost us as long as we own them, either in maintenance or storage. When we have too many things, we no longer own them—they own us.

Simplifying our lives with fewer things will save not only our energy, as we've seen, but also our money, money that can be put into retirement or other savings—not used to buy more stuff.

The most difficult part of getting control of our finances is getting control of our own impulses and desires. Companies are brilliant at coming up with products they know will appeal to us, things we'll find nearly impossible to resist. Then they hire advertising firms who know us better than we know ourselves when it comes to subtle ways of getting us to buy their products.

The most devastating to our finances are not the big-ticket items, though we get suckered into buying too many of those, too. The worst assault on our finances are the smaller things, things under fifty or one-hundred dollars. All those ten-dollar and twenty-dollar items that we can pay for with pocket cash. All those times we buy fast food for lunch instead of packing a lunch. All those cheap knickknacks, cute items, and tacky doo-dads that appeal to us, but that we really don't need. Consider the shopping malls where we pick up ever more accessories, more outfits, more shoes—all on sale! Look at how much we saved! No. Look at how much we spent. Did we need the shoes? Were the old ones worn out? Were we replacing accessories that were several years old and worn? Probably not.

We each know our own weaknesses, what we like to buy. What we need to pay attention to is how those buying habits drain our finances and how quickly they add up over time. Take a five-dollar fast-food lunch twice a week for a year (though most Americans eat out more often than twice a week). That's 520 dollars. Buying half that many lunches would save 260 dollars. When was the last time you were in a pinch and could have used an extra 260 dollars? If you eat out twice a week, you can honestly say you didn't have the extra cash because you ate it. What's more, the fast food you bought negatively affected your health. In this case, cleaning up one bad habit can give you double the return—a healthier body and healthier finances.

Obviously, cutting back fast food won't fund your retirement, unless you eat out nearly every day. Our point is this: look at all the little things you spend money on and then question why you're getting those items. Do you really need them, or is there a cheaper way to accomplish the same goal? Are you being driven by what your really need? Or, are you being driven by wants? Are you indulging desires created by a culture of consumerism? Are you buying things to feel accepted or to fit in with those around you?

Once again, the key to gaining control and simplifying our finances is being honest with ourselves and paying attention to the habits we have. It doesn't take a financial planner to figure out you'll be better off putting money in the bank instead of in your pocket.

Family and Friends

Though we love them, hold them dear, and may want to be with them, family and friends can place expectations and demands upon us that unnecessarily complicate our lives. These relationships can be a major source of conflict and distress. The solution? Move across the country, or to another country, and cancel your long-distance service. Let them call you, but always let the answering machine get the phone. Eventually they'll quit calling. Of course, we're just kidding! (Or are we?!)

Adult Children

One of the greatest sources of stress is the underlying tension and conflict between parents and their adult children. Few parents seem to transition easily into letting their kids become adults in their own right. And let's face it: some parents are never able to see their adult children completely as adults. Forty-year-old executives are scolded like school kids when visiting "home" for the holidays. Then parents wonder why the "kids" don't come over often for a visit.

Other family dynamics from long-standing family behavior patterns or cultural or ethnic family values may create similar tensions. The expectations family places upon us may be enormous—and onerous—but we're culturally expected to have "family values" and are made to feel guilty if we fail to meet all the spoken and unspoken expectations. These problems have created no end of material for stand-up comics, movies, and TV sitcoms. We all recognize the plight of trying to juggle all the in-laws and their feelings about the holidays. Promoted as the time of love and peace, the holidays turn out to be anything but for many families. We may still love our families, but they very likely complicate our lives. What to do? How do you reclaim your own sanity without making the whole family hate you?

For parents with adult children, our advice is pay attention to how you speak to or treat your grown children. Are you saying the same kinds of things to them now that you were when they were teenagers? Do you use the same tone of voice? Are your adult children reluctant to come see you? You may need to reconsider how you're interacting with them. Do you give unsolicited advice? Here's a good rule of thumb: if your adult child doesn't ask for advice, don't give it. Simply enjoy their company and treasure the time they spend with you. Bite your tongue to hamburger if you need to, if you think they're making a mistake. If, and when, they want your advice, they'll ask. They may appreciate you more for not offering. If, and when, they do make a mistake, you won't need to tell them about that, either. Keep quiet about the whole thing, and you'll win *major* parent points. Many parent-adult child relationships could be healed if parents tried to listen more, advise less, and judge less. Unsolicited advice creates resentment when your son or daughter feels that you're treating them like a child. This includes a judgmental tone of voice and withholding of approval.

For adult children of parents who still treat you like a child, we're sorry, but there's little you can do to change your parents' behavior. So, change what you can in them, but also change what's going on *between your ears*. A reframed attitude about parents can do a lot for your sanity.

Romance

If you've followed all of our other advice, you should have more time for romance. The problem is, many of us carry overly-romanticized ideals of spontaneous romantic interludes. We mistakenly think romance should be as perfect, luxurious, and intense as an ad for champagne. When we set our expectations so high, the only possible result is disappointment. As unromantic as it may sound, we recommend lowering expectations to reasonable levels and planning ahead for romance.

Even if you think that advice "ruins" everything, stay with us here. First, challenge where your notions of romance come from. Women in particular are taught through cultural messages to expect the moon—that is, a perfect moonlit night, with a perfect gown, a chauffeured limousine, flowers, with wining and dining. It's the image of the perfect prom night. We associate luxury—and expense—with romance.

We contend, however, that if the relationship is what it should be, the focus should be on the relationship itself, on your partner and yourself, not on the surrounding luxuries. Sure, those things are nice and add to the atmosphere, but they may also add unneeded expense and financial stress. What have you gained with a romantic evening if two weeks later you're arguing about the credit-card bills?

In a world of consumerism and affluenza, it's all the more important to find ways to learn to cherish one another rather than getting caught up in all the things that are supposed to make an evening romantic. Personally, we rebel against Valentine's Day, with all its commercial demands and all the silly clutter sold in its name. We prefer surprising each other with unexpected cards or flowers—a simple bouquet of carnations or daisies—at other times of the year. We enjoy each others' company and find everyday ways to be together, whether it's routine walks with the dogs, regular shopping trips for needed items, or something as mundane as washing the truck. The focus is on the time together and the conversation we have, not on wild and unreasonable expectations of the perfect evening out.

Certainly we believe in couples taking time for a night on the town—don't get us wrong. But that's not the only option, nor always the best option for romance. In our experience, the couples with long-lasting, successful relationships are those in which the partners find everyday ways to enjoy and take time for one another.

In Conclusion

We *choose* the complexity level of our lives. Certainly some is inescapable in a modern, technologically driven world, but much of what complicates our lives is of our own doing and choosing. In trying to have it all or do it all for ourselves, the irony is we may lose the very thing we're trying so hard to satisfy: ourselves. But we do have a clear choice to say *no* to demands and opportunities, to people, to our own unchecked wants. Therein lies the path to simplicity and ultimately to more energy.

FEATURE:

DON'T WORK HARDER—JUST BETTER

George describes himself as a incurable workaholic. Nothing makes him happier than to work twelve hours a day, juggle multiple projects, function in different careers, and work at the computer until late at night. However, when he does this, he quickly gets out of balance and starts to suffer the consequences. At the top of the list of these are not spending enough time with Christie or enough time in spiritual pursuits. Fortunately, he does somehow find time to eat well, exercise everyday, and take care of himself. Unfortunately, he's clearly addicted to working. (While we resist applying the term "addiction" to all instances of excessive behavior, it does seem to fit with work—though not quite in the same way as drug addiction or alcoholism.)

Workaholism is a condition that many psychologists see as a serious problem—but one that's also socially accepted. Many companies expect their employees to be more than dedicated to their careers. Modern corporate culture rewards goal-directed, motivated employees with promotions, more money, and awards—not to mention the prestige that accompanies worldly success.

Complicating matters, the United States has, on average, the lowest rates of vacation and sick leave for employees in the industrialized world. Every other comparable modern nation and economy allows its workers more time off. Our nation was founded on the fundamental idea of the Puritan Work Ethic, where a person's value is established through what and how much he or she does rather than valuing who he or she is. If we find ourselves feeling obligated to work harder, or feeling guilty for not working hard enough, or feeling like we've never put in enough hours, we're accurately reflecting the culture in which we live. It's no accident that a culture so prone to workaholism is also a culture with insatiable consumerism and entertainment. One extreme creates the appetite for the other. Sanity lies in breaking the cycle.

Before blaming everything on power-driven bosses, let's first take an honest look at our working day. One cause of needing to work extra hours is office socializing. How often does a quick conference on a work item transform into a fifteen-minute personal conversation? No doubt we need good interpersonal relationships with coworkers, and we can develop positive relationships in the work place. But these relationships and personal conversations need to be kept carefully in check. One fifteen-minute conversation per day adds up to over sixty-two hours per year. That's a week and a half of work lost to idle conversation.

One of the best ways to control wandering conversations is to gracefully bow out with comments like, "This is interesting, but I have to get back to my project in order to meet the deadline. How about you tell me about this over lunch tomorrow?" In other words, keep personal conversations to personal time. Not only will your boss love you for it, but you'll be more productive and less stressed.

Another strategy is to avoid the initial conversation to start with. We know the people who are office talkers. Find out when they usually go to the copier, get coffee, or run errands. Leave items for them in their "in-basket" or on their desk with a note. Usually this accomplishes the same task and avoids the risk of your getting caught up in unproductive conversation.

Another strategy is using voice- and e-mail. When we leave messages, we're more likely to get right to the point: we want to type as little as possible, and voice-mail systems cut off long messages. These keep us focused on the essential work to be done. Christie found that in her office, when the company adopted an internal e-mail system and she used it instead of memos and running to talk to people, her productivity went up by 25 percent, and she spent far fewer days working extra hours.

Yet another strategy is closing your office door or putting up a "Please do not disturb" sign at your cubicle. These signs should include notes of when you'll be available. This puts people on notice that you're focused on a project, but will answer their questions when you're available. This streamlines your time and gets more work done.

Some might argue that these strategies are antisocial. To a certain extent, that's the point. You don't have to be unkind or rude, but first you're obligated to give your employer a full day's work. Second, what is the logic in spending time socializing during the day, only to have to work extra hours? Would you rather be spending time with your coworkers, or be on your own time at home with your family?

We believe life and stress in the workplace can be more easily controlled by managing access to your time. Certainly this doesn't solve all the workplace stresses, and you may need to consider alternative employment and career opportunities. But if you're struggling to get your work done in a reasonable amount of working hours, we challenge you to consider how productive your time really is. Simplifying your work may be a matter of reducing idle conversation. Likewise, we also challenge you to apply the other simplification strategies of this chapter to your workplace.

PART 3

THE SPIRIT AND EVERYDAY ENERGY

CHAPTER 9

NURTURE YOUR SOUL

The wealth of the soul is the only true wealth.

—Lucian

In these final two chapters of *Stop Feeling Tired!*, we want to address *spirituality*, or religious belief and practice, as an aid to finding life balance and overcoming fatigue.

Interestingly, the spiritual side of life is far too often ignored in our busy society, as well as in self-help psychology books. Why? Busy people don't always want to invest the time or put forth any effort to work on their spiritual development. Instead, it's easier to take medications, spend more money, accumulate clutter, and socialize in what amounts to an empty attempt to fill their spiritual void.

In our view, true balance and energy can't be found without simultaneously working on one's spirituality. It's at the heart of all we do! Unfortunately, neither of us knows a great deal about religious expressions other than our own. We're both life-long Christians, so we'll be discussing spirituality mostly from that perspective.

Some might argue with our using "spirituality" and "religion" in the same breadth. Granted, many people distinguish between the two:

spirituality referring to inner devotion and religion referring to institutional trappings. And we'd agree that the two are not really the same. For example, self-help groups like Alcoholics Anonymous (AA) emphasize teaching people how to reach spiritual heights by acknowledging their dependence on a "Higher Power" without necessarily attending a church, synagogue, or mosque. But for many people, the two concepts go together; they're inseparable. We know many, many people who experience great comfort and closeness to God within organized religion. They've found it necessary to be a part of a larger faith group in order to progress in their spiritual life. So, we don't want to leave you with impression that everyone who tries to be more spiritual is absolutely a card-carrying, tithing member of any particular group. Many are, but many aren't. In this chapter, although we acknowledge the potential differences between the "spiritual" versus the "religious," we'll use these terms synonymously for convenience.

Over the years we've studied and practiced both formal and informal spiritual practices, a few of which we humbly share with you in the following pages. Not all have involved our going to church. Yes, we enjoy being part of the larger faith community and sharing in fellowship with other like-minded folks. But some days we get much more out of walking our dogs and enjoying nature than listening to "just try harder" preaching. Other days we have stimulating talks about God that surpass any Bible study we've ever attended. The good news here is that God neither lives in a box nor expects us to. *There's room for both formal and informal spiritual and religious practice.* This means it's okay that our desire for God finds expression in different ways. Some people need to be very vocal in their worship and prayer, while others need to be quiet and reflective. Regardless of what works best for you, the idea is to do what it takes to grow in your relationship to God and your fellow human beings. This, in turn, will help you find what Christianity refers to as the *virtue of temperance*: the kind of balance that leads to sane, healthy, and energetic living in all areas of your life.

Spirituality and Psychology

Spirituality is crucial to our human need to discover meaning and purpose in life. Whether our spirituality involves active and formal membership in a religious organization or a more personal and independent approach, growing spiritually makes us keenly aware of the deeper aspects of life. It helps us develop a desire and capacity for vision, purpose, and values. It helps us have ethics and morals that shape our lives. And, most importantly, it helps us love others and our planet while, at the same time, we become closer to God.

Clearly, spirituality is important and satisfying to most of us, which explains why so many psychologists and sociologists have also shown an eager interest in the topic. In fact, research studies have repeatedly shown how spirituality and mental health are positively related, indicating that the more spiritual you are, the more likely you'll have a healthy psyche and satisfying life. And when this happens, you can't help but feel more love and zest for life.

A good deal of evidence suggests that spiritual practices improve mental health in many ways. From our experience, regular spiritual practice can:

- Improve your self-esteem while reducing your anxiety and depression

- Contribute to helping you develop sound moral judgment and ethical principles

- Increase your marital stability, happiness, and satisfaction

- Contribute to helping you avoid the perils of inner-city poverty, such as crime, delinquency, and substance abuse

- Help you overcome various social problems, including divorce, suicide, alcohol and drug abuse, crime, pornography, and unintended pregnancies

- Enhance your physical health by increasing longevity and lessening the incidence of serious diseases

- Improve your chances of recovery from a serious illness

How does all of this work? Besides God's role in our lives, researchers believe spirituality and religious practice positively influence the way you cognitively process life events. Restated simply, *having a spiritual frame of mind helps you make sense of the world around you.* We suppose you could label this a type of spiritual reframing. And when you can reframe you life from a spiritual perspective, you're in a better position to reverse the effects of stress and imbalance. Or, in equation form:

spiritual reframing → more calm → more balance → more energy

That said, let's take a look at a few basic spiritual practices that, when combined with other techniques described in this book, can help you feel more grounded, balanced, and energetic.

Freedom From Materialism

Few would argue that to focus on spiritual matters requires at least some detachment from the world. From a Christian perspective, spiritually-minded people have always been called to live in the world without being a part of the world (John 17:13-16). (We know this sounds paradoxical, but that's what mysteries are all about, right? Such apparent paradoxes and dilemmas stretch our imaginations and give us food for thought.) At a practical level, what this means is you're better off letting go of the worldly baggage that keeps you from growing spiritually. Anything that gets in the way of your walk with God should be discarded when the time is right. Notice we said "when the time is right." If you give away all your belongings, quit your job, and move to a mountain before you're ready, you'll be miserable and probably regret what you've done. Yes, the lighter a wheel rolls, the faster it'll move forward. But a wheel that's completely off the ground won't move forward at all. See our point? *Extremes do little to help you find balance and energy.*

While not possible for most of us, certain persons throughout history have exercised a special God-given gift to remove themselves more fully from the world. For example, around the middle of the second century, many Christian men and women decided to their raise their personal consciousness and standards of holiness by practicing poverty, fasting, prayer, chastity, and celibacy for the sake of God. Later, around the middle of the third century, Christians began retreating from the world and into the desert (in order to leave the world in a greater way), where they established permanent places to live.

Perhaps the best example of such a person was Saint Anthony the Great, who left his worldly life around the year 285 to reside in the Egyptian desert. St. Anthony is often considered the founder of Christian monasticism, and a great many people have followed his example over the centuries. His primary means of increasing spirituality was contemplative prayer, a version of which we'll describe below. Of course, giving up a materialistic life doesn't belong only to Christianity. Most spiritual disciplines endorse loosening one's load in this world as a means of becoming closer to God and devoting more energy to the welfare of others. Consider the life of India's Mahatma Gandhi, whose nonmaterialism and selfless dedication to the poor has proven to be an enduring inspiration to us all. The point here: the lighter your baggage is, the easier and faster you'll move forward. Just remember, though, to take it easy. To overlighten your load is to cause yourself needless stress and exhaustion. To reiterate, spiritual extremes in either direction don't promote balance. So, remember to practice the "Three R's": be *rational, reasonable,* and *reserved*.

Prayer and Meditation

Some form of prayer is the basis of a spiritual life—the source of our experiencing God and the higher aspects of life. Plain and simple, prayer involves your talking to God (and hopefully listening to God, too!). It doesn't matter how or where you talk to God, it's still prayer. A friend of George's even claims he does his most intense praying while in the bathroom!

Meditative Prayer

How few of us spend time in prayer of any depth. If we did, the world would clearly be a better place. For most of us, though, prayer means little more than a few words at the dinner table or reciting mechanical prayers while standing or kneeling in a religious service. In order to enter more deeply into the life of prayer, our religion (Eastern Orthodoxy) recommends the "Jesus Prayer," or "Prayer of the Heart." It goes like this: "Lord Jesus Christ, Son of God, have mercy upon me a sinner." Of course, you can change the words to fit your own belief system and tradition. The point here is the prayer is repeated over and over again, almost like a mantra, to help you focus your thoughts onto spiritual matters. Indeed, such contemplative prayers as the Jesus Prayer are a form of Christian meditation.

Sadly, we do get flack from some Western Christians when we use the word "meditation," which they associate with "heretical," "non-Scriptural," or "pagan" religious practices. The word derives from the Latin *meditatio*, which translates as reflection, contemplation, rehearsal, and practice. It carries no religious connotation. In its original meaning, to mediate is to reflect on something important. As one personal example, we like to mediate on how thankful we are for all the daily blessings we enjoy.

Intercessory Prayer

An absolutely fascinating literature has recently developed describing the power of *intercessory prayer*, or praying for the welfare of others. In particular, scientists have developed an interest in whether prayer can improve the health of those for whom prayers are offered. Perhaps the best documented experimental study to examine this question was a 1988 study of intercessory prayer conducted at San Francisco General Hospital. The study found that prayer benefitted patients in that these people were able to go home from the hospital sooner (Byrd 1988). Specifically, Byrd studied patients who entered that hospital's coronary-care unit. Subjects were randomly assigned to two groups, and the intercessors were only given their patient's first name and health problem. Patients in the experimental group were prayed for, while patients in the control group weren't. Using a double-blind experimental design (meaning that neither doctor's nor patients knew who was praying or being prayed for), Byrd found statistically significant differences between the prayed-for group and the control group. In other words, patients who were prayed for, overall, improved more than patients who weren't prayed for. Although this and similar studies have attracted their share of both supporters and critics, keep in mind Byrd's research results appeared in the well-respected, doctor-reviewed *Southern Medical Journal*.

In short, prayer can bring many benefits to your life, including helping you achieve spiritual balance. And it can help you help others. As you become accustomed to daily prayer and contemplation, you'll experience deeply moving consolation. That's when you'll be closer to clarity of thought, spiritual peace, benevolence toward your neighbors, and thankfulness to God.

Silence and Solitude

Silence and solitude are time-honored spiritual techniques for quieting the mind and listening to the subtle voice of God. Why do we need these? Think about it. We're constantly besieged by noise from the minute we rise in the morning until we go to sleep at night: televisions, radios, traffic jams, cars honking, people pulling at us, and the daily hullabaloo at work or school. And if this weren't bad enough, our minds race all day long about every urgency imaginable with the voices of all the *gotta's* and *have to's* urging us on, so much so that sometimes we can't even hear ourselves think. Our question: where's peace of mind in all of this? When do we have time to be still and listen to God as well as our own inner self?

Silence and solitude can be an important answer. You can't effectively pray, meditate, or read the spiritual literature of your religion without first removing the clutter of noise, whether it's external, internal, or both. The Bible tells us that even Jesus had to escape the crowds and find time alone to spend in prayer (Luke 5:16). If Jesus needed to do this, then how can the rest us presume we don't have to do likewise?

We're convinced that the distractions of everyday life sabotage our becoming closer to God, finding balance, and feeling good. That's why we find it helpful to take time during the day—even if only a couple of minutes at our desk, in the car, or wherever—to be alone and quiet. We highly recommend this simple approach for ridding your mind of useless clutter.

Fasting

In chapter 3, we talked about the importance of fasting for physical balance. Now we'd like to briefly remind you of the importance of fasting for spiritual balance. Fasting helps purify your spiritual sensitivity. It also helps you change the way you think about yourself, let go of undesirable habits, and reflect on how fortunate we Americans are to have plenty of food and drink. Fasting is also a time-honored spiritual practice intended to quiet your mind's critical voice and obsession with food and other material objects.

Spiritual fasting accomplishes two basic goals. First, it breaks your body's hold over your will and emotions. Second, it demonstrates just how accustomed you've become to having your way. In other words, fasting frees your soul by breaking up the daily habits and patterns upon which you've become so reliant. And when your "pleasure patterns" are thwarted, your body isn't satisfied, and you're left dependent on your own inner resources. This is an interesting space in which to find yourself.

Of course, any form of fasting—which can range from absolute abstinence (water only) to strict dietary changes (for example, no meat)—should only be done under the direct supervision of a physician or other health-care practitioner.

Reflective Reading and Writing

We love nothing better than to enjoy a quiet, cozy day reading uplifting books and articles. We find cool, cloudy, and rainy days to be our favorite. George likes having a large mug of flavored coffee, along with classical music quietly playing in the background, while he ponders life's greatest moments. Christie reads and reflects while listening to quiet new-age music and sipping on herbal tea.

Books have a special way of touching our spirits. And we're not talking about computerized e-books or PDF files! While there's certainly a place for electronic books and other such media, when it comes to spiritual reading, we like to hold a real book. Handling the cover, turning the pages, and closing the book for a few moments to contemplate—we've simply never found an adequate substitute. In a way, our reading rituals allow us to feel in touch with the book's author and personalize whatever message is being communicated to us.

Christie also finds writing in a journal a very useful spiritual tool. Journaling gives her an opportunity to gather her thoughts, think about deeper issues, and express herself. It also allows her an opportunity to solve problems and set more realistic goals. Finally, she uses spiritual journaling as a written record of her personal responses to spiritual matters.

Learning From a Spiritual Teacher

Finally, many seekers of truth find value in studying under a spiritual teacher or director. The spiritual life is always best realized within a *relationship*, in this case, between a "directee" and a director, teacher, elder, Father confessor, or other spiritual mentor. The process usually includes detailed teaching provided by the spiritual director, such as instruction in the ancient art of prayer, guided reading and study, and exercises in focusing inner attention. Spirituality often includes ascetic bodily practices (for example, simple living, abstinence and fasting, increased attendance at worship services, tithing) that complement such prayer and study. All of this is intended to challenge a person's physical senses and energies in order to learn control and discipline—essentials in the journey to personal awareness and service to God and neighbor.

Spiritual direction has been an important feature of Eastern Orthodoxy for a long time. A few highly spiritual persons, in circumstances where guidance was unavailable, were able to receive spiritual direction via lifelong prayer and study of sacred writings. Many found the wasteland of the Middle-Eastern desert to be the ideal location to gain some distance from the distractions of life and search the depths of their hearts. Today, the process can seem more like a counseling session between director and directee. Still, the mystical nature of personal spirituality (the "inner way") manages to come through. Consider these words from Joseph Allen, author of *Inner Way: Toward a Rebirth of Eastern Christian Spiritual Direction* (1994):

> The director initially works to push the directee "back on himself," bringing him to face his inner being, to see what is

there, what is operating, what is true. To travel the *inner way* means to allow the light of discernment, about which St. John Cassian spoke, to probe the depths of one's heart and mind. The elder's function is to guide the person into the places where such discoveries can be made because light has newly shined upon them. And what does he hope the directee will see? Again, both his *motivation* (perception) and his *behavior*, which together constitute a person's life (25).

In Conclusion

Modern science has historically avoided the study of spirituality, entrusting the topic to theologians and philosophers. Yet the role of spirituality in human wellness can't be ignored. Increasing numbers of studies are confirming what spiritually-minded people have known for ages: *spirituality restores balance and positively influences both physical and emotional health.* Indeed, the inner peace that faith imparts enables us to respond more effectively to life's hurdles by providing a sense of purpose and guidelines for living. Many of us turn to our spiritual convictions when we're face with difficult situations. In doing so, we're better able to counteract our sense of helplessness, find order in our life circumstances, and cope with whatever ails us—be it exhaustion, stress, sickness, or anything else.

Finally, perhaps the most striking aspect of spirituality is the fact it deals in the here and now. No matter what method or expression is chosen, spirituality is the way in which we express our faith and serve in the world. It is the sum total of the attitudes and actions that define our existence and nurture our soul.

FEATURE:

TAI CHI AND QIGONG

We'd like to mention two "active" Asian exercises for finding balance and energy. Although these could've easily been included in chapter 4, we're mentioning them here because of these practices' unique spirit-balancing properties.

In addition to herbs and acupuncture, Chinese medicine (TCM) utilizes, among a myriad of techniques, the internal martial arts known as *Tai Chi* (*Taijiquan*) and *Qigong* as spiritual exercises to achieve balance of mind, body, and spirit. Both of these "soft style" martial arts (versus "hard style" techniques like *Kung Fu*), as they are practiced today in the West, can be thought of as active, moving forms of meditation and yoga. Many of the movements were first described based on the natural movements of animals, although in *Tai Chi* and *Qigong* they are performed softly, serenely, and slowly.

Here are two of George's favorite *Qigong* exercises.

Polishing the Bass Drum. In this exercise, you imagine a large bass drum in front of you, with the skinny part of the drum facing your torso. Stand with your feet comfortably apart and with left foot in front of your right. You move the palms of your hands in circular fashion (clockwise) along the skin of the imaginary drum. In other words, the drum is mentally placed between the palms of your hands. As your hands move away from you, you shift your balance onto your left foot, which is forward; as your hands move back toward you, you shift your balance back onto your right foot. Do this thirty times very slowly, exhaling when your weight is on your left foot, and inhaling when it's on your right. Repeat the exercise, now starting with your right foot in front.

Polishing the Sky Mirror. In this exercise, you imagine a large, round mirror facing the sky. Stand with your feet comfortably apart, about shoulder's width. You move the palms of your hands in circular fashion (clockwise) along the horizontal surface of the imaginary mirror. When your hands are in the middle of the mirror, your weight is equally distributed between both feet. As your hands move to the left, you shift your balance onto your left foot; as your hands move to the right, you shift your balance back onto your right foot. Do this thirty times very slowly, inhaling and exhaling as your weight shifts from foot to foot.

CHAPTER 10

FIND MEANING AND PURPOSE

*But the fruit of the Spirit is love, joy, peace, patience,
kindness, goodness, faithfulness, gentleness, self-control.
Against such there is no law.*

—Saint Paul

In our brief final chapter of *Stop Feeling Tired!*, we explore several of the deeper issues of life. Our hopeful aim is to help you think about your life and see more clearly why you're on this earth.

Why Am I Here?

At one time or another, most of us ponder the great question of earthly life: "Why am I here?" But engaging this question in a real sense takes time, motivation, and effort. Sadly, few of us are willing to do this. And that's why most of us never truly come to terms with the reasons for our existence. We run hurriedly from one appointment to the next. We schedule too many activities. We seclude ourselves from others to keep from letting our inner selves be known. We do whatever we can to avoid being authentic. After all, it's easier to run from ourselves than face ourselves.

In psychology, the *existential-humanistic perspective* emphasizes the importance of your immediate experience, self-acceptance, and self-actualization. These three qualities of existence lay the groundwork for helping us find meaning and purpose in life, which in turn help us find balance and love.

Immediate Experience

Being aware of the here and now is an important aspect of living a balanced life. Psychologically speaking, you can't effectively interact in the world unless you have insight into your present self, into what makes you tick today—your feelings, your motives, your desires, and your dreams.

If you're not in touch with the here and now, you're likely either stuck in the past or hung up on the future. The most common emotions associated with these two sides of the same coin, respectively, are anger and anxiety. And these emotions, as we learned in chapter 5, can generate all kinds of undesirable behaviors. For example, if you can't (or won't) get over the hurdles from your childhood (and we all have them!), you'll experience anger—or one its cousins, depression or guilt—that you can't seem to control. You'll find yourself obsessing over things people said or did years or even decades ago. To try to feel better, you might lash out at the people originally responsible (if they're still around) or at others who had nothing to do with your woes. Unfortunately, none of this does any good. We're not saying it's wrong to feel anger and express it. It's our opinion that a rational and measured response of anger, when appropriate, is healthy. But continuing to get mad (or depressed or guilty) over events that have long since passed will only interfere with your ability to handle today's problems. There comes a time to move on, to toss out all of the skeletons hanging in the closet of your past.

Then there's anxiety over what *might* happen. We've addressed catastrophizing in earlier chapters, but want to take a moment here to remind you that it does little good to fret about what could happen to you. Eastern philosophers often speak of how futile it is to worry about a tiger that might cross your path in the jungle. Yes, we all know that life is full of dangers. And if your common sense tells you danger is near, then by all means defend yourself! But there's no point cowering and hiding under the covers "just in case" when you have no good reason to believe harm is just around the corner. Go about your business, live in the moment, think rationally, and do your best to avoid getting hurt.

In short, focusing too much on the past or the future detracts from the present, and this can be a cause of stress, imbalance, and lack of energy.

Self-Acceptance

Being self-accepting can do much to promote calm and self-fulfillment in life. Self-acceptance means acknowledging your own existence and your right to live happily. It also means loving yourself and being content with who you are *today*. You might refer to this as self-love or self-esteem, but regardless of how you label it, self-acceptance is a major first step to improving your life. It's your pact with yourself to accept, support, validate, and cherish who you are right now, even though you realize areas of your life probably leave some room for improvement.

Why don't we accept ourselves? All too often, we seek absolute approval from those around us instead of finding approval within ourselves. And when we don't receive it, we end up rating ourselves by putting ourselves down. There really is a better way: appreciate your existence and, if necessary, rate what or how you're doing, but resist rating yourself as a person.

Another factor in not accepting ourselves is fear of going stagnant. Many of us believe self-acceptance means thinking we don't need to make any changes. And so the logic goes: if we accept ourselves the way we are, we'll go stale and never try to improve ourselves. Rest assured, life simply doesn't work this way! Human beings are never stagnant; we're always growing, changing, and adapting. And we all have behaviors we'd like to do something about—none of us is perfect. Yes, it's okay to accept ourselves just as we are today while at the same time acknowledging we have behaviors, thoughts, and emotions that we want or need to change.

Self-acceptance is actually a first step in the process of change. Ordinarily, we rate our entire being as bad with the hope it'll motivate us to make changes. Again the logic goes like this: if we feel bad enough about ourselves, then hopefully we'll transform ourselves into someone better. Does this work? Not really. This type of irrational thinking does little else than deplete our energy and keep us from experiencing life in the fullest sense. The negative thinking works in direct contrast to what we want. So, if you experience everyday tiredness, learning to accept yourself as you are can do much to bring back your lost zip.

Self-Actualization

The same can also be said of self-actualization, or becoming your very best. Realizing your inner potential, expressed in every area of life, can help you feel rejuvenated. How? If you're a self-actualizing type, you probably enjoy a certain comfortable relationship with your life that shows itself in everything you do. You take responsibility for yourself and refuse to blame others for your misfortunes. You take risks, don't worry about unknowns, and like to use your reason and logic to make sense out of the senseless. And you don't let your unhappy childhood experiences get you down today. In other words, to be self-fulfilling is to be rational and balanced, which means you'll have greater enthusiasm and energy to face whatever comes your way.

This isn't to imply that a self-actualizing person has no imperfections or problems. Quite the contrary, you're painfully aware of your own flaws, yet you're joyfully aware of your own growth processes. You also understand that there aren't any magic wands that can be waved over your head to change you. But by working, practicing, planning, and steadily acting, you can stay rational and then deal with most any life hurdle, including stress and chronic fatigue.

What's It All About?

Many people find the answer to this question through a combination of inner work and service to others. This is also an essentially spiritual question; therefore, the answer must be essentially spiritual, too.

The spiritual life is always realized within a context of relationships. Whether encountering one's neighbor or God, the spiritual life doesn't exist—can't exist—within a vacuum. How, then, is the average person to apply spirituality, realize meaning and purpose in life, and follow a spiritual life in today's modern and complicated world?

In the midst of economic and racial inequalities, when large numbers of us are in mental, physical, and spiritual need, when evil conditions continue to exist unabated, *change begins in the heart but is expressed in our relationships.* This concept of *faith* and *service*, or "vocation" to others, is to see the inherent *mysterion* ("mystery") of those relationships. Faith and service to God, neighbor, and the planet certainly differs from a purely social program involving legal persuasion that compels people to do what's right. Instead, our faith and service are our *response* to God and all the blessings that we enjoy in this life.

Humility, Inner Life, and Spirituality

Before a vocation to action can take form, inner change is necessary. Central to the entire process of spiritual formation is *humility*, the inner realization that we need a Higher Power. It's also the realization of our need to be modest, loving, and trusting in our thoughts, bodies, and spirits. Humility, then, existentially accompanies us in our life's spiritual journey through such acts as love, charity, patience, relatedness, empathy, respect, contentment, gratitude, and virtue—to name only several. Of course, these inward and outward expressions of humility and service are but a small part of having a spiritual life; flowing from our inner depths, these are a beginning, not an ending unto themselves.

Sadly, many average Americans believe they're leading a first-class spiritual life solely as a result of weekly worship attendance and financial contributions. While these activities are certainly rewarding, they don't automatically demonstrate an actual change of heart, only membership in a religious organization. If you truly desire to lead a spiritual life, you first need to examine your own inner life, your own inner depths. *Only when the inner self is confronted can we reach out to others with pure intention.* And only in this place can we find lasting spiritual healing.

In short, an active spiritual life is much more than an awareness of social inequalities or desire to do good. It's our *reply*—an action that manifests itself as nothing less than an earnest attempt to live out our life's mission.

In Conclusion

If you're searching for meaning and purpose in your life, you're in good company. All of us want to understand the larger significance of our existence. Let's face it, without a sense of meaning, day-to-day life becomes empty and tiresome.

Having a mission in life is to think and act, to do and be, to become our very best. Purpose prompts us to seek out what is true, just, moral, and beautiful. It prompts us to use our God-given reason to find moderation, harmony, and stability in ourselves. It helps us live as we're designed to live. And most importantly, it connects us to the Higher Power who created us.

The spiritual life is a rich way of living that shows us our purpose. As you develop spiritually, you might find your purpose is to have a particular manner of being in the world that permeates your entire life—caring for the needy, being honest, showing courage in the face of calamity, living simply, and standing up for the underdog. Or, you might find your purpose is to serve the world through volunteering, creating art, loving your children, or practicing any of a million seemingly little acts that are, in fact, so important. The key here is: *spirituality leads to purpose that leads to an inner life that leads to action.*

Some critics might argue that the spiritual life is too demanding for the average person. Nothing is further from the truth! Remember, Jesus expounded the many great truths of mercy and grace to the simple and unlearned common folk of that day. He taught at the people's level, "where they were at," so to speak.

And this is precisely the same place where we listen, learn, and find answers to our deepest questions about life.

FEATURE:
ON A RESOLUTE AND
SUSTAINED PURPOSE

For our final quote in *Stop Feeling Tired!*, we'd like you to consider these insightful words on beginning a new life from Tito Colliander's classic text on Eastern spiritual mysticism and faith, *Way of the Ascetics: The Ancient Tradition of Discipline and Inner Growth* (1960):

Faith comes not from pondering but through action. Not words and speculation but experience teaches us what God is. To let in fresh air we have to open a window; to get tanned we must go out into the sunshine. Achieving faith is no different; we never reach a goal by just sitting in comfort and waiting, say the holy Fathers.

However weighed down and entangled in earthly fetters you may be, it can never be too late. Not without reason is it written that Abraham was seventy-five when he set forth, and the labourer who comes in the eleventh hour gets the same wages as the one who comes in the first.

Nor can it be too early. A forest fire cannot be put out too soon; would you see your soul ravaged and charred?

No, this moment, the instant you make your resolution, you will show by your action that you have taken leave of your old self and have now begun a new life, with a new destination and a new way of living (1–2).

Epilogue

In these pages, we've talked to you about balancing your body, mind, and spirit. We've challenged you to transform your thinking and life-style, live simpler, live healthier—all as your personal route to more energy. Take a moment now and reflect on everything we've said so far. Maybe flip back through the pages and remind yourself of the highlights. Do you see a pattern? A theme? We hope so.

When it comes to regaining energy, balancing our lives, and feeling better about ourselves, much of it comes down to one thing: *choice*. We really *do* have the power to choose. We can choose a calmer, simpler, more balanced life that brings us more energy and positive feelings about ourselves and our lives. We can listen to the voice of reason and ignore the unrealistic demands of an ever-faster world. We can live healthier, happier, more energetic lives.

Admittedly, there are things in life beyond our control. A loved one with chronic illness or aging family members are some of life's possible challenges that we can't control. But the truth is, most of what ails us is well within our control—we simply have to make it happen. And when we control those things, the uncontrollable events are more manageable.

When our lives feel out of control, disorganized, and we feel tired, we can take the steps to organize, to rethink our situations. The hardest part about making those choices is sticking to them. Think about it: if the choices were easy and the follow-through effortless, we wouldn't have the problem in the first place. Right? While the solution may not always be easy, and while we're all fallible, the route to more energy is clearly doable. The only thing stopping us, the *only* thing between us and more energy, more full living, is ourselves. We don't have the energy we want because we haven't done what it takes to go after it. Our inertia feeds itself.

All it takes is for you to choose to start doing things differently. Be honest with yourself. Examine and challenge your thinking. Transform your thinking. Simplify your life. Make plans and set goals to do what you know you need to do in terms of eating right and being active.

You can continue to live the stressed-out, tired life, the life that caused you to pick up this book in the first place—or you can live the life of your choice. You can live a life driven by hectic demands and chaos or one actively engaged in living motivated by your own sufficient energy.

Here's the reality: all of us only get one walk through life, and it's a short journey at that. We don't see this as discouraging, but as a challenge, as a motivator to go forward and do our best for ourselves—not selfishly, but in a manner that supports our own endeavors. Life is far too short to waste with stress, undue complexity, and lost energy. We want the vitality every moment has to offer, and that comes through making the choices that bring us energy.

Who wouldn't want an energetic life, lived the way you want to live it? Who wouldn't want peace of mind and peace with yourself? Who wouldn't want a healthy, balanced body, mind, and spirit? Who wouldn't want to feel good? Who wouldn't make that choice?

Contact Us

In the final analysis, everyday tiredness can be an uncomfortable problem, but it needn't get the best of you. Readied with the information and techniques presented in this book, you can overcome exhaustion and regain control of your life! We truly hope the information and resources contained in *Stop Feeling Tired!* help you to find freedom from your chronic tiredness.

While everyday tiredness presents a definite challenge to millions of Americans, healing is possible. And you've taken that all-important first step toward recovery by reading this book. May you find the life answers that you're looking for, as well as lasting freedom from whatever stresses, unrealistic thoughts, and unhealthy habits haunt you.

Of course, we hope you've enjoyed reading *Stop Feeling Tired!* and that you've gained at least a few new insights. Although we can't promise to answer your letter, we'd like to hear from you concerning any impact that this book has had on your life. Feel free to contact us through our publisher at the following address:

George and Christie Zgourides
c/o New Harbinger Publications
5674 Shattuck Avenue
Oakland, California 94609

Please accept our best wishes as you pursue freedom from exhaustion!

Resources

Here's a helpful listing of holistic health, nutritional, mental health, medical, and spiritual resources for your use:

Albert Ellis Institute
45 East 65th Street, New York, NY 10021
800-323-4738
Internet: www.REBT.org

American Counseling Association
5999 Stevenson Avenue, Alexandria, VA 22304
703-823-9800
Internet: www.counseling.org

American Chiropractic Association
1701 Clarendon Boulevard, Arlington, VA 22209
800-986-4636
Internet: www.amerchiro.org

American Institute for Cognitive Therapy
136 East 57th Street, Suite 1101, New York, NY 10022
212-308-2440
Internet: www.cognitivetherapynyc.com

American Massage Therapy Association
820 Davis Street, Evanston, IL 60201
847-864-0123
Internet: www.amtamassage.org

American Psychiatric Association
1400 K Street N., Washington, DC 20005

888-357-7924
Internet: www.psych.org

American Psychological Association
750 First Street, NE, Washington, DC 20002
800-374-2721; 202-336-5500
Internet: www.apa.org

Anxiety Disorders Association of America (ADAA)
11900 Parklawn Drive, Suite 100, Rockville, MD 20852
301-231-9350
Internet: www.adaa.org

Association for Advancement of Behavior Therapy (AABT)
305 Seventh Avenue, 16th Floor, New York, NY 10001
212-647-1890
Internet: www.aabt.org

Council of Colleges of Acupuncture and Oriental Medicine
7501 Greenway Center Drive, Suite 820, Greenbelt, MD 20770
301-313-0868
Internet: www.ccaom.org

Emotions Anonymous International
P.O. Box 4245, St. Paul, MN 55104
651-647-9712
Internet: www.mtn.org/EA

National Institute of Mental Health
6001 Executive Boulevard, Room 8184, MSC 9663, Bethesda, MD 20892
800-64-PANIC; 301-443-4513
Internet: www.nimh.nih.gov

National Mental Health Association
1021 Prince Street, Alexandria, VA 22314
800/969-NMHA; 703-684-7722
Internet: www.nmha.org

Additional Web sites:

> http://odp.od.nih.gov (Office of Disease Prevention)
>
> http://www.health.gov/dietaryguidelines (USDA's Nutrition and Your Health: Dietary Guidelines for Americans)
>
> http://www.nal.usda.gov (National Agriculture Library)
>
> http://www.OrganizedHome.com (OrganizedHome.com)

RECOMMENDED READING

Accolla, D., and P. Yates. 1996. *Back to Balance: A Holistic Self-Help Guide to Eastern Remedies*. New York: Kodansha International.

Austin, M. D. 1997. *The Healing Bath: Using Essential Oil Therapy to Balance Body Energy*. Portland, OR: Healing Arts Press.

Bloom, A. 1970. *Beginning to Pray*. Mahway, NJ: Paulist Press.

Castleman, M. 2000. *Blended Medicine: The Best Choices in Healing*. New York: Rodale.

Cooper, S. 2000. *Fibromyalgia and Chronic Fatigue: Acutherapy and Holistic Approaches*. Ogden, UT: Life Circles Publications.

Cousens, G., and D. Wagner. 2000. *Tachyon Energy: A New Paradigm in Holistic Healing*. Berkeley, CA: North Atlantic Books.

Cruise, J., and A. Robbins. 2001. *8 Minutes in the Morning: A Simple Way to Start Your Day That Burns Fat and Sheds the Pounds*. Emmaus, PA: Rodale Press.

Davis, B. 1990. *Monastery Without Walls: Daily Life in the Silence*. Berkeley, CA: Celestial Arts.

DeMarco, T. 2001. *Slack: Getting Past Burnout, Busywork, and the Myth of Total Efficiency*. New York: Broadway Books.

Eden, D. 1999. *Energy Medicine: Balance Your Body's Energies for Optimum Health, Joy, and Vitality*. New York: J. P. Tarcher.

Gerber, R. 2000. *Vibrational Medicine for the 21st Century: The Complete Guide to Energy Healing and Spiritual Transformation.* New York: Eagle Brook.

Henner, M. 1998. *Marilu Henner's Total Health Makeover: 10 Steps to Your B.E.S.T. Body: Balance, Energy, Stamina, Toxin-Free.* New York: Reganbooks.

Jacobson, M. F., and J. Hurley. 2002. *Restaurant Confidential.* New York: Workman Publishing Company.

McGee-Cooper, A. 1992. *You Don't Have to Go Home from Work Exhausted! A Program to Bring Joy, Energy, and Balance to Your Life.* New York: Bantam.

Mills, B., A. Ross, and M. L. Blasutta. 1997. *Desperation Dinners!* New York: Workman Publishing Company.

Nelson, M. M., and M. Nelson. 2001. *Stop Clutter from Stealing Your Life.* Franklin Lakes, NJ: New Page Books.

Prout, L. 2000. *Live in the Balance: The Ground-Breaking East-West Nutrition Program.* New York: Marlowe and Company.

Schechter, H. 2000. *Let Go of Clutter.* New York: McGraw Hill.

Skelly, M., A. Helm, and P. Brown. 1999. *Alternative Treatments for Fibromyalgia and Chronic Fatigue Syndrome: Insights from Practitioners and Patients.* Alameda CA: Hunter House.

St. James, E. 1998. *The Simplicity Reader.* New York: Smithmark.

Teitelbaum, J. 2001. *From Fatigued to Fantastic!: A Proven Program to Regain Vibrant Health, Based on a New Scientific Study Showing Effective Treatment for Chronic Fatigue and Fibromyalgia.* New York: Penguin Putnam.

REFERENCES

Allen, J. J. 1994. *Inner Way: Toward a Rebirth of Eastern Christian Spiritual Direction*. Grand Rapids, MI: William B. Eerdmans Publishing Company.

American Psychiatric Association. 2000. *Diagnostic and Statistical Manual of Mental Disorders*. 4th ed., Text rev. Washington, DC.

Antony, M. M., and R. P. Swinson. 1998. *When Perfect Isn't Good Enough: Strategies for Coping with Perfectionism*. Oakland, CA: New Harbinger Publications.

Balch, P. A., and J. F. Balch. 2000. *Prescription for Nutritional Healing*. 3rd ed. New York: Avery.

Beck, A. T. 1979. *Cognitive Therapy and the Emotional Disorders*. New York: Meridian.

Burns, D. D. 1999. *The Feeling Good Handbook*. Rev. ed. New York: Plume.

Byers, T., M. Nestle, A. McTiernan, C. Doyle, A. Currie-Williams, T. Gansler, M. Thun, and the American Cancer Society 2001 Nutrition and Physical Activity Guidelines Advisory Committee. 2002. American Cancer Society guidelines on nutrition and physical activity for cancer prevention: Reducing the risk of cancer with healthy food choices and physical activity. *CA: A Cancer Journal for Clinicians* 52(2):92-119.

Byrd, R. C. 1988. Positive therapeutic effects of intercessory prayer in a coronary care unit population. *Southern Medical Journal* July:826-829.

Callahan, M. 2002. Deconstructing the Subway Diet. *Cooking Light.* Jan./Feb:30.

Carlson, R. 1997. *Don't Sweat the Small Stuff . . . and It's All Small Stuff.* New York: Hyperion.

Center for Food Safety and Applied Nutrition, U.S. Food and Drug Administration. 2002 (March). *Kava-Containing Dietary Supplements May Be Associated with Sever Liver Injury.* Rockville MD: Available at http://vm.cfsan.fda.gov/~dms/addskava.html

Chapman-Smith, D. 2000. *The Chiropractic Profession.* West Des Moines, Iowa: NCMIC Group Inc.

Chappell Cain, A., Ed. 1999. *Cooking Light 5-Ingredient 15-Minute Cookbook.* Birmingham, AL: Oxmoor House.

Colliander, T. 1960. *Way of the Ascetics: The Ancient Tradition of Discipline and Inner Growth.* New York: Harper and Row.

Ellis, A. 1962. *Reason and Emotion in Psychotherapy.* New York: Lyle Stuart.

————. 1988. *How to Stubbornly Refuse to Make Yourself Miserable About Anything—Yes, Anything!* Secaucus, New Jersey: Lyle and Stuart.

Ewer, C. T. E. 2002. *A Tightwad's Guide to Getting Organized.* Available at http://organizedhome.com/time/tightwad.html

Fransen, J., and I. J. Russell. 1996. *The Fibromyalgia Help Book: Practical Guide to Living Better with Fibromyalgia.* Saint Paul, MN: Smith House Press.

Gruenwald, J., T. Brendler, and C. Jaenicke, Eds. 1998. *PDR for Herbal Medicines.* Montvale, NJ: Medical Economics Company.

Hoffman, R. L. 1993. *Tired All the Time: How to Regain Your Lost Energy.* New York: Poseidon.

Jason, L. A., J. A. Richman, A. W. Rademaker, K. M. Jordan, A. V. Plioplys, R. R. Taylor, W. McCready, C. F. Huang, and S. Plioplys. 1999. A Community-Based Study of Chronic Fatigue Syndrome. *Archives of Internal Medicine* 159(18):2129-2137.

Kuntzleman, C. T. 1992. *Maximizing Your Energy and Personal Productivity: A Nationally Renowned Health Expert Shows How to Unleash Your Energy Potential for a More Healthy, Productive, and Satisfying Life.* Chaska, MN: Nordic Press.

Lazarus, A. A., and C. N. Lazarus. 1997. *The 60-Second Shrink: 101 Strategies For Staying Sane in a Crazy World.* San Luis Obispo, CA: Impact Publishers.

Lazarus, A. A., C. N. Lazarus, and A. Fay. 1993. *Don't Believe It For A Minute: Forty Toxic Ideas that are Driving You Crazy.* San Luis Obispo, CA: Impact Publishers.

Levey, J., and M. Levey. 1998. *Living in Balance: A Dynamic Approach for Creating Harmony and Wholeness in a Chaotic World*. Berkeley, CA: Conari Press.

Linde, K., and M. Bemer. 1999. Commentary: Has hypericum found its place in antidepressant treatment? *British Medical Journal* 319:1539.

Luhrs, J. 1997. *The Simple Living Guide: A Sourcebook for Less Stressful, More Joyful Living*. New York: Broadway Books.

Maciocia, G. 1994. *The Practice of Chinese Medicine: The Treatment of Diseases with Acupuncture and Chinese Herbs*. London: Churchill Livingstone.

Mallinger, A. E., and J. DeWyze. 1992. *Too Perfect: When Being in Control Gets Out of Control*. New York: Clarkson Potter Publishers.

Mann, F. 1973. *Acupuncture: The Ancient Chinese Art of Healing and How It Works Scientifically*. New York: Vintage Books.

National Institute of Diabetes and Digestive and Kidney Diseases (NIDDK). 2002. *Statistics Related to Overweight and Obesity*. Bethesda, MD: National Institutes of Health/U.S. Department of Health and Human Services.

National Institutes of Health. 1997. *Acupuncture: NIH Consensus Statement Online* 15(5):1-34. Bethesda, MD: National Institutes of Health. Available at http://odp.od.nih.gov/consensus/cons/107/107_statement.htm.

National Institute on Aging (NIA). 2002. *Exercise: Feeling Fit for Life*. Bethesda, MD: National Institutes of Health/U.S. Department of Health and Human Services.

Sarno, J. E. 1991. *Healing Back Pain: The Mind-Body Connection*. New York: Warner Books.

Schlosser, E. 2002. *Fast Food Nation: The Dark Side of the All-American Meal*. New York: HarperCollins.

Seyle, H. 1976. *The Stress of Life*. New York: McGraw-Hill.

Tappan, F. M. 1988. *Healing Massage Techniques: Holistic, Classic, and Emerging Methods*. 2nd ed. East Norwalk, CT: Appleton and Lange.

Troiano, R. P., C. A. Macera, and R. Ballard-Barbash. 2001. Be physically active each day. How can we know? *The Journal of Nutrition* 131(2S):S451-S460.

United States Department of Health and Human Services. 1992. *Healthy People 2000: National Health Promotion and Disease Prevention Objectives: Full Report with Commentary*. Washington, DC.

Ware, T. 1997. *The Orthodox Church*. London: Penguin.

Wolpe, J. 1958. *Psychotherapy by Reciprocal Inhibition*. Stanford, CA: Stanford University Press.

STOP FEELING TIRED!

About the Authors

George D. Zgourides, Psy.D., is a clinical psychologist and clergyman specializing in mind-body psychology, spiritual issues, and integrative approaches to healing. He is the author and coauthor of numerous books, including *Stop Worrying About Your Health!* and *Shy Bladder Syndrome.*

Christie Zgourides, M.A., is a medical practice executive at Pathology Consultants of New Mexico in Roswell, an online adjunct faculty member at Kaplan College in Boca Raton, Florida, and a former associate professor at Warner Pacific College in Portland, Oregon.

Some Other
New Harbinger Titles

Responsible Drinking, Item DRINK $18.95

The Mitral Valve Prolapse/Dysautonomia Survival Guide,
Item MVPS $14.95

Stop Worrying Abour Your Health, Item SWYH $14.95

The Vulvodynia Survival Guide, Item VSG $15.95

The Multifidus Back Pain Solution, Item MBPS $12.95

Move Your Body, Tone Your Mood, Item MBTM $17.95

The Chronic Illness Workbook, Item CNIW $16.95

Coping with Crohn's Disease, Item CPCD $15.95

The Woman's Book of Sleep, Item WBS $14.95

The Trigger Point Therapy Workbook, Item TPTW $19.95

Fibromyalgia and Chronic Myofascial Pain Syndrome, second edition,
Item FMS2 $19.95

Kill the Craving, Item KC $18.95

Rosacea, Item ROSA $13.95

Thinking Pregnant, Item TKPG $13.95

Shy Bladder Syndrome, Item SBDS $13.95

Help for Hairpullers, Item HFHP $13.95

Coping with Chronic Fatigue Syndrome, Item CFS $13.95

The Stop Smoking Workbook, Item SMOK $17.95

Multiple Chemical Sensitivity, Item MCS $16.95

Breaking the Bonds of Irritable Bowel Syndrome, Item IBS $14.95

Parkinson's Disease and the Art of Moving, Item PARK $16.95

The Addiction Workbook, Item AWB $18.95

Call **toll free, 1-800-748-6273,** or log on to our online bookstore at **www.newharbinger.com** to order. Have your Visa or Mastercard number ready. Or send a check for the titles you want to New Harbinger Publications, Inc., 5674 Shattuck Ave., Oakland, CA 94609. Include $4.50 for the first book and 75¢ for each additional book, to cover shipping and handling. (California residents please include appropriate sales tax.) Allow two to five weeks for delivery.

Prices subject to change without notice.